T0073757

WITHIN REASON

Within Reason

A Liberal Public Health for an Illiberal Time

SANDRO GALEA

The University of Chicago Press

CHICAGO AND LONDON

The University of Chicago Press, Chicago 60637
The University of Chicago Press, Ltd., London
© 2023 by The University of Chicago
Published 2023
Printed in the United States of America

32 31 30 29 28 27 26 25 24 23   1 2 3 4 5

ISBN-13: 978-0-226-82291-4 (paper)
ISBN-13: 978-0-226-82886-2 (e-book)
DOI: https://doi.org/10.7208/chicago/9780226828862.001.0001

Library of Congress Cataloging-in-Publication Data

Names: Galea, Sandro, author.
Title: Within reason : a liberal public health for an illiberal time / Sandro Galea.
Description: Chicago : The University of Chicago Press, 2023. |
    Includes bibliographical references and index.
Identifiers: LCCN 2023006596 | ISBN 9780226822914 (paperback) |
    ISBN 9780226828862 (ebook)
Subjects: LCSH: Public health—Political aspects—United States. | Public health—
    Social aspects—United States. | COVID-19 (Disease)—United States—
    Influence. | Liberalism—United States.
Classification: LCC RA445 .G352 2023 | DDC 362.1962/4144—dc23/eng/20230428
LC record available at https://lccn.loc.gov/2023006596

♾ This paper meets the requirements of ANSI/NISO Z39.48-1992
(Permanence of Paper).

This book is dedicated, as always, to
Isabel Tess Galea, Oliver Luke Galea,
and Dr. Margaret Kruk.

CONTENTS

INTRODUCTION

One of my weekend traditions is to go running each Saturday morning when I'm in my hometown of Brookline, Massachusetts. On the way home, as a reward for the exercise, I typically stop at my favorite bakery to pick up pastries. In winter 2022, when I finished a run I saw a note on the bakery door: "While we know the indoor mask mandate has been lifted in Brookline, we will continue to require a mask to shop . . . until further notice." It struck me as remarkable that the bakery proprietors presumably knew the town had consulted public health professionals when making the decision to lift the mask mandate and that the policy was supported by science. What's more, Brookline is home to many medical professionals owing to the proximity of world-class hospitals in the Boston area, so they should have felt assured that the public health advice given to town leaders was first-rate. It's likely the bakery owners did not themselves consult any public health professionals when choosing their own masking policy, because any professionals familiar with the data would probably have advised them to let masking remain optional, as the city had done. The notice thus conveyed a revealing subtext. It effectively said, "The owners of this establishment are aware that public health experts have concluded the science no longer supports the need for mandatory masking in settings like this. However, we are choosing to ignore this guidance because we fundamentally distrust public health experts. We prefer to follow our instincts and ask you to do the same."

This speaks to an enormous loss of faith in the public health establishment, a direct result of mistakes made during COVID-19. Brookline, Massachusetts, is one of the most politically progressive places in the country. During the pandemic, public health directives often met with much more compliance in places like this than in more conservative regions—at least that was the perception. Yet the owners of the Brookline bakery clearly did not have enough faith in public health officials to follow their advice on masking. Or perhaps they were in fact disposed to believe the advice of public health but took the course they did out of fear or to signal their allegiance to a political and cultural in-group. Either possibility reflects failure by public health officials. Consider this question: Would such a note on the bakery door even have been conceivable before the pandemic? Can anyone recall an instance before COVID when a business establishment put a note on its door that said, effectively, "We realize that health experts have decreed X, but we ask you to observe Y"? To my mind, that such a notice may have seemed unremarkable in 2022 reflects an enormous loss of respect for the stature of public health experts and should call for honest self-reflection. If the public health establishment is not believed because officials are thought to be dishonest or incompetent, this is a self-evident problem, and we should ask ourselves why such a perception might have taken hold. If we are believed, yet our advice is ignored because the extreme embrace of restrictive public health measures—going beyond even the advice of epidemiologists—has become, above all, a political and cultural signifier akin to the red hats worn by some supporters of former president Donald Trump, we should likewise ask ourselves what role we might have played in bringing this about.

This book attempts to address that question. Has the public health establishment contributed to the way the bakery sees its advice? The more I have thought about this question, the more I have found that is troubling about the evolution of public health over the past few years.

Let me start by offering three recent examples: During the Trump years, many people working in public health criticized the Centers for Disease Control and Prevention (CDC) for engaging in what looked like politically motivated behavior. In December 2017, for example, the *Washington Post* published a report claiming that CDC officials had apparently been banned from using certain words in their budget documents, words that included *fetus*, *diversity*, and *transgender*. This sparked an outcry among many in public health and on the political left. (The CDC director later said no words were banned at the organization.) The response to this perceived censorship reflected public health's wariness of the CDC's deviating from what had been its nonpartisan, science-based work of promoting good health. This wariness was captured by a 2020 *STAT News* article, "The CDC has always been an apolitical island. That's left it defenseless against Trump."

But the CDC has seldom been apolitical, and public health's pushback on CDC's engagement with politics has been rather one-sided. As an illustration, consider the CDC's engagement with mask wearing in 2021, during the Biden administration. On May 13, 2021, the CDC announced that people who were fully vaccinated against COVID no longer had to wear masks indoors or outdoors. An email obtained through a Freedom of Information Act request shows that, the next day, the White House director of labor engagement reached out to the CDC chief of staff to ensure coordination between the CDC, the Biden White House, and the leaders of the National Education Association—the teachers' union. This was not the only time the CDC was shown to have worked with teachers' unions to shape health guidance. The American Federation of Teachers also communicated with CDC and Biden White House officials on school reopening guidelines, with the union at one point even suggesting language for the CDC's guidance on reopening schools. This politicizing of the CDC did not, as far as I could see, arouse any criticism from within public health.

Now let's look at a moment when public health *did* rise in protest. In fall 2020, a group of epidemiologists and academics signed what became known as the Great Barrington Declaration. The declaration advocated an approach to COVID that aimed to minimize the social and economic harms caused by widespread lockdowns. It called for a "focused prevention" strategy in which those most at risk—older adults and those with underlying health conditions—received protection, while those at minimal risk would no longer be subject to strict lockdowns. The goal was to reach herd immunity while acknowledging the elevated risk faced by certain segments of the population and working in accordance with the data to protect the vulnerable. While much about the proposal was supported by our understanding of the virus at the time—and, indeed, remains so by our subsequent knowledge of both the disease and the harmful effects of lockdowns—it makes sense that such a recommendation would be subject to rigorous debate. What is perhaps surprising is the level of vitriol it sparked from many in the media and the public health community. The declaration was called "ill-advised and arrogant" and "an ethical nightmare," and it was accused of giving "oxygen to fringe groups."

As a third example, let us consider, perhaps controversially, public health's insistence in the United States on the importance of vaccinating very young children against COVID. Before going further, I should here state that, after careful thought, I chose to vaccinate my own kids, and I do not regret the decision. However, it is worth noting that, as soon as vaccines were available, many in public health argued that we could be sure the vaccines were largely safe and that any negative effects were certainly outweighed by the danger of kids remaining unvaccinated. Yet this was not obviously true. The danger posed by COVID varied significantly by age, with young children at low risk. And while the data largely supported the view that the vaccines were safe and effective, we were not in a position to give assurances about their long-term risk profile because these data did not yet exist. These considerations are particularly relevant when we are imposing vaccines on children, a group that was never really at substantial risk from COVID. Fundamentally, we wanted to vaccinate children because it protected us adults. And that should have been the subject of mature conversation. Nevertheless, anyone who raised these concerns faced a chilly reception within the US public health community and in the larger progressive spaces within which public health is nested. This response contrasted with other places like the United Kingdom, where the conversation about whether to vaccinate children was more open and robust.

It is possible to read these stories and be completely untroubled by them. It is possible, for example, to think that it is right for the CDC to issue ostensibly science-based guidance that in fact emerged from consultation with special interests. One might feel that the Biden White House and the teachers' unions were on the right side of the masking debate and that their collaboration with the CDC reflected evenhanded stewardship of the issue. It is possible to favor aggressive pushback against the Great Barrington Declaration, perhaps because the declaration was embraced by some on the right as justification for less stringent lockdowns. And it is possible to think that those who raised any form of skepticism about vaccines during the pandemic deserved to face similar pushback.

Yet to be untroubled by all this is to overlook—or even endorse—certain worrying trends within public health. The common thread linking the anecdotes I've shared is that each reflects a challenge to the liberalism that has long been the animating principle of our field. Consider the politicizing of the CDC. The work of the CDC never has, and never should have been, entirely apolitical. Insofar as politics is about the allocation of resources, much of public health—which is also about the allocation of resources—is political. It then strikes me that public health's criticism of the CDC's politicizing under Trump was transparently self-serving and hypocritical. This was made abundantly clear when we in the field turned a blind eye to the clear collaboration between the CDC and the teachers' unions under President Biden. But we criticized the former, not the latter. To be clear, I'm not sure I object to the CDC's working with partners in executive, legislative, or other branches of government. What does trouble me is when political bias causes us to cherry-pick what we criticize, reflecting how we as a field have been co-opted by partisan politics, leading us to neglect our core values when that seems to be in the interest of our "side."

This partisan dynamic was also reflected in the response to the Great Barrington Declaration. At times the backlash sounded more like religious fundamentalists denouncing heresy than like scientists soberly engaging with the pros and cons of an argument. I should note that I do not agree with the declaration's conclusions. I didn't agree with them then, and I don't agree with them now. Yet I would not deny that the reasoning behind some of the declaration reflects several sound epidemiological principles— indeed, the concept of herd immunity could be said to be Epidemiology 101. Aligning our response to a virus with our understanding of its relative risks is likewise elementary to the work of public health. It is an approach that the CDC would eventually embrace as it became clear that COVID would likely be with us for some time. While the sum total of the declaration may have been problematic, the response to the document was, I would argue, much worse for what it reflected about the intersection of public health and the hyperpartisan era in which COVID emerged. During the pandemic, discussion of mitigation measures based on relative risk rather than on indefinite, societywide lockdowns was often met by a tone of opposition that those of us who were used to sober, evidence-based discussion found striking. Such a tone is not consistent with the way public health has long conducted itself. But it is consistent with the behavior of a political interest group engaged in partisan conflict. And that's a problem.

It's likewise a problem to see a chilling of free and open debate about something as important as vaccinating children during a pandemic. Of course some would argue that it is precisely because it was during a pandemic that the COVID moment was not the time for such conversations, and that the crisis made such debate tantamount to causing physical harm. Yet it is not having these debates that undermines trust in science in the long term. It is pretending we know when we might not that results in bakeries' taking scientific matters into their own hands. Science should never be afraid of the truth, or of the rigorous debate that gets us to it. And it is antiscientific to claim we know what cannot be known—the long-term effects of a brand-new vaccine. The conversation about vaccinating children also reflects our unwillingness to grapple with the trade-offs inherent in choices about health policy. All of this raises ethical questions: Were we pushing to vaccinate children for their sake or for ours? Were we doing it to support health or to make a political point?

Whatever these examples are, they do not reflect the liberalism that once defined public health. I have worked in public health for over twenty years. I joined the field because I believed in its power to create a healthier world. I believed the public health community had this power because it was united around certain core values. Centrally, these values are freedom of speech and debate, adherence to the scientific method, and an embrace of diversity—diversity of identity and diversity of thoughts and opinions. These values enable us to generate ideas, correct for error, and work together toward the common good.

These values are not unique to public health. They are the foundation of a liberal society. I should clarify at the outset what I mean by "liberal." I do not mean liberal in the sense of being left-wing or politically progressive. I mean liberal in the broader sense. We in the United States have inherited a system with roots in the European Enlightenment, a time when societies began to organize around reason, free speech, the pursuit of truth, and the preservation of liberty. Out of these values emerged liberal democracy and modern science. I am aware that liberalism in its wider sense can mean many things to many people. I use the word "liberal" to mean the core values I have described, leaving it to others to apply different uses to the word in the context of different arguments.

For years I've had reason to think myself a public health insider. I have been privileged to work within leading public health institutions, I have collaborated with colleagues from all over the world, and I have traveled extensively as part of my work. I've seen public health up close for most of my professional life, but I no longer recognize what I see. This book, then, emerges from something of an identity crisis as I find myself feeling like an outsider in a field I've long considered home.

My personal identity crisis was precipitated by a real crisis: the COVID pandemic. During COVID, public health did much to rise to the occasion and safeguard health. But it also in many ways succumbed to the temptation to lean toward illiberalism. This was perhaps inevitable. The pandemic was a moment when public health received more attention and power than it had ever had in the United States. While we were often able to leverage our newfound status toward a more effective pursuit of our work, at times this new prestige went to our heads. This caused us to do what human beings often do when we receive a windfall: we forgot where we came from. Namely, we forgot the liberal values that used to be the basis of all we did.

My goal for this book is to help us see where and why we have gone astray and to begin to chart a course back to a liberal public health, one that regains the trust of the populations—and the bakeries—we serve. The chapters of this book are based on columns I wrote for my weekly online newsletter, *The Healthiest Goldfish*, during the COVID pandemic. In keeping with the online roots of these chapters, the book is structured as a series of essays rather than as one continuous argument. In making the case for a liberal public health policy, they touch on many subjects, including public health's engagement with economics, race, class, politics, bureaucracy, freedom, tradition, speech, objectivity, and history. The book thus is a mosaic of the issues facing our field and their intersection with the effort to restore a liberal public health policy. The book is divided into sections. The first, "Foundations," features reflections on the structural forces that shape health and on how these forces have at times been shaped by the illiberalism of this moment. The second, "Heresies," touches on several topics that contemporary public health has found it hard to discuss in recent years, but that are nevertheless core to supporting a healthier world. The third section, "Hopes," details emerging positive trends that could help us find our way back to a liberal version of public health. A final section, "In Conclusion," gives some thoughts on the road ahead.

Although the topics in these sections are eclectic, they are organized around a vision for a liberal public health based on our engagement with the central problems of this moment. To my thinking, public health faces five key obstacles to a full restoration of its liberal ideals. I list them here as an anchor to the reflections contained in these chapters.

1. SCIENCE AND PUBLIC HEALTH INSTITUTIONS HAVE BECOME POLITICIZED

In recent years, public health's alignment with left-wing politics has become increasingly explicit. This was perhaps understandable as a reaction to the right-wing authoritarianism and antihealth policies of former president Donald Trump. However, it led to public health's being perceived by many—for reasons fair and unfair—as a mere adjunct of progressive politics, and specifically of the Democratic Party. To the extent that our science and institutions may indeed have been co-opted by ideology, we need to reform our engagement with politics so as to ensure that our advice to policymakers and the public reflects a process of reason and analysis rather than political expedience.

2. WE HAVE FORGOTTEN OUR ROOTS

Public health emerged from a tradition of scientific inquiry that had its roots in the European Enlightenment, a period that also birthed the political liberalism we have inherited. This tradition prizes freedom of speech and thought, reasoned methodology, and the pursuit of truth as the basis for a better world. It is opposed to oppressive ideology—on both the left and the right—and to institutions that codify habits of mind that are inimical to freedom. Over time this tradition has done much to help create—haltingly, imperfectly—a better world. In pursuit of this world, we have in recent years risked trading what has worked for a vision of progress that rests on illiberal foundations. Such a vision can seem to promise quicker results but, as I will argue in this book, is ultimately self-defeating. When we forget our roots, or willingly diverge from them, we risk undermining our science and our effectiveness as advocates for a healthier world. I note that an effort to reclaim roots does not entail forsaking progress. There is much to lament about the principles of the Enlightenment and much to learn from other philosophical traditions. But that learning is better served by a robust engagement with what has already served us well than by a wholesale repudiation of it.

3. WE HAVE BECOME POOR AT WEIGHING TRADE-OFFS

During COVID, we embraced widespread lockdowns of social and economic life as a means of slowing the spread of the virus. As these lockdowns continued, they took a significant toll on our economy, our education system, and our mental and physical health. Yet even as the evidence of these consequences became clear, those who suggested a more measured approach to lockdowns were vilified by many in public health. This reflects an underdevelopment of our ability to weigh trade-offs in our thinking about what is good for health. When we lack this ability, we are liable to slip into zero-sum thinking about the policies that shape health, causing us to misstep, and even to do harm.

4. MEDIA FEEDBACK LOOPS HAVE BECOME THE NEW PEER REVIEW

Peer review is a means of testing our scientific conclusions to ascertain their integrity and support better scholarship. In recent years, forms of media have begun to take the place of peer review in shaping the trajectory of our thoughts. Peer review continues, of course, but far more influential in some ways are the feedback loops enforced by media bubbles and social media platforms like Twitter, where public health practitioners are rewarded for expressing ideas that fall within certain ideological parameters and punished for straying outside them. Where peer review helps sharpen our pursuit of truth, the media often amplifies distorted or incomplete thinking, undermining the intellectual foundations of our field.

5. WE HAVE PRIORITIZED THE CULTIVATION OF INFLUENCE OVER THE PURSUIT OF TRUTH

During the pandemic, public health experts were granted unprecedented influence. We had the ear of policymakers, we helped shape guidance that affected the lives of billions, we saw our profiles elevated in the media. It would be hard for anyone to be unaffected by such a sudden rush of prestige. This is perhaps why public health officials took actions during COVID in which the evidence-based pursuit of health was often secondary or incidental to maintaining our continued influence. We saw this in our willingness to toe an ever-shifting party line, and when called out we could say we were just "following the science." We saw it in the way many of us closed ranks around the Biden administration when it came to power. We saw it in our difficulty in criticizing public health institutions, which are the source of much bureaucratic influence but are also the locus of much that needs reform. The pursuit of political and bureaucratic influence has come at the expense of the pursuit of truth—of our capacity to follow the science wherever it leads, to speak the truth about our institutions, and to criticize leaders even when they are on our "side." What is ironic about this is that the more our pursuit of influence caries us away from our core mission of promoting health, the less substance there is to what we communicate to the public. This causes us to lose influence with our core constituency— the populations we serve—diminishing trust in public health and trading our capacity to support health over the long term for the sugar high of momentary relevance and prestige.

These are obstacles indeed to a liberal vision of public health. Fortunately it is well within our power to correct them, to shape a better future for our field and for the populations we serve.

Speaking as I do from within public health, I think I can anticipate some of the criticisms this book will receive. Let me address them here. A core criticism will likely be that I have forsaken the progressive values that animate public health, that I have gone right wing. This is nonsense. Far from changing my views, I see myself as being consistent. I have always identified as a progressive, pursuing a healthier world by working to improve the social, economic, and political conditions that shape health. In this pursuit I have advocated for a range of progressive policies, some of which could be characterized as radical. They include Medicare for all, universal basic income and a generous social safety net, reparations for slavery, liberal immigration policies, and commonsense gun safety reform. Indeed, my criticism of contemporary public health has little to do with policy. There is room within liberalism for all kinds of policy interventions, from the radical to the reactionary. That is the virtue of a liberal system: it is flexible and can accommodate a wide range of views within a framework of empiricism, open debate, and democratic decision-making. It is only when we move toward dismantling the norms and values that keep this system robust that it becomes necessary to draw a line. While we may think casting aside liberalism will bring us closer to our policy goals, in the end we will have undercut the very conditions that enable progress. And we have made much progress. Injustices and inequities persist and should continue to be addressed. But when we compare the progress that has emerged from post-Enlightenment liberalism to the rest of human history, we see an extraordinary era of social and political improvement. It is as a progressive who values this achievement and recognizes its fragility that I wrote this book.

Another likely criticism is that it is somehow inappropriate to point out illiberalism in left-leaning public health when illiberalism on the right has become so egregious in the Trump era. In fact, I see illiberalism on the left as an extension of the broader deleterious effects of Trump. I have often felt that much of what we have seen in public health, and within progressivism more broadly, has been a reaction to Trump's election. The elevation of such a figure to the presidency seemed to confirm the worst narratives about our country. This put much of public health on something akin to war footing, as we hunkered down in our ideological camps, sealed ourselves off from complicating nuance, and accepted the necessity of behaving in ways that reflect battlefield conditions rather than the norms of liberal discourse. This reflects how opponents of Trump, perhaps ironically, can find themselves behaving like him, discarding liberal norms as a response to his influence. His ability to corrupt the actions of well-intentioned people is one of his more pernicious contributions to the present moment.

Faced with the trauma of the Trump era, public health's response is entirely understandable. Liberalism is easily tarred as milquetoast, inadequate when confronted with an empowered right wing and the legacy of racism, xenophobia, and misogyny it often exploits. With the clear and present threat coming from the other side of the political divide, is now really the time, one might ask, to point fingers at the excesses of progressivism? This question is an example of a long-standing rhetorical dodge known as bothsidesism. The argument that we should ignore our own challenges for fear of empowering our opponents—whose flaws may well be worse than ours—is old and potent. It is also wrong. If we ignore the ways we are falling short because we do not wish to help our foes, we simply help them in a different way—by making ourselves weaker through our inability to speak freely, self-correct, and think for ourselves. This does no favors for the populations we serve. Here is George Orwell writing in 1944:

> A phrase much used in political circles in this country is "playing into the hands of." It is a sort of charm or incantation to silence uncomfortable truths. When you are told that by saying this, that or the other you are "playing into the hands of" some sinister enemy, you know that it is your duty to shut up immediately.
>
> For example, if you say anything damaging about British imperialism, you are playing into the hands of Dr. Goebbels. If you criticize Stalin you are playing into the hands of the *Tablet* and the *Daily Telegraph*. If you criticize Chiang Kai-Shek you are playing into the hands of Wang Ching-Wei—and so on, indefinitely.
>
> Objectively this charge is often true. It is always difficult to attack one party to a dispute without temporarily helping the other. Some of Gandhi's remarks have been very useful to the Japanese. The extreme Tories will seize on anything anti-Russian, and don't necessarily mind if it comes from Trotskyist instead of right-wing sources. The American imperialists, advancing to the attack behind a smoke-screen of novelists, are always on the look-out for any disreputable detail about the British Empire. And if you write anything truthful about the London slums, you are liable to hear it repeated on the Nazi radio a week later. But what, then, are you expected to do? Pretend there are no slums?

The temptation to ignore or downplay the illiberal turn taken by public health in the face of even greater illiberalism on the right is strong. But doing so would be tantamount to, in Orwell's phrase, pretending there are no slums. This would violate the spirit of public health. Our mission has always been to face the conditions that shape health and to tell the truth about them, even when doing so upsets the status quo. We should do no less when considering the state of our own field. I am opposed to illiberalism wherever it emerges, whether on the right or the left, within the Trump White House or the CDC. There are, of course, clear and important differences between these two entities, and I do not mean to compare them in any fundamental way. I submit this provocative juxtaposition only to make the point that while illiberalism can be different in scope, it is not different in kind. The impulse toward illiberalism is the same wherever it appears. Recognizing this impulse within ourselves is necessary to prevent illiberalism from becoming our defining feature rather than a temptation we occasionally succumb to.

Core to doing so is ensuring that public health remains informed by a diverse range of perspectives. Part of our liberal inheritance is our capacity to give a hearing to many different ideas without fear that doing so will seem like endorsing a particular side. We can hear all sides of a debate without conceding that they are morally equivalent, just as we can remain open to many ideas while being selective about which ones we embrace. Core to liberalism is the proposition that such conversations are the best way to test the integrity of our thinking. The more robust the debate, the better the chance of our emerging from it stronger, sharper.

I am aware that much of what is in this book may be hard for those in public health to hear. I am also aware that many friends and colleagues may disagree with my view of public health's current trajectory. Nevertheless, I wrote this book because I believe the values that animate public health matter. Part of our strength is our capacity to disagree, to have debates, to pursue reason wherever it leads. We are most effective when our loyalty is to data, and to the core principles that animate us, not to ideology. We are most influential not when we are aligned with politicians in power or when a crisis invests us with bureaucratic sway, but when the public trusts us. That trust depends on whether they believe we are honest brokers. If we are not making a good faith effort to follow the data, if we seem to suppress information because it is politically inconvenient, if we appear to wield power for its own sake, we diminish our field. Public health is too important for us to let that happen. Our task is nothing less than creating a healthier world. Accomplishing it will take a liberal public health, not an ideologically compromised shadow of our former selves. I called this book *Within Reason* because I believe public health can function only within a context of reason. This means renewing our commitment to the liberal values that have helped us come so far. To create a better world, we need to be at our best. This book aims to help us get there.

SOURCES

Applebaum, A. "The New Puritans." *Atlantic*, August 31, 2021. https://www.theatlantic
.com/magazine/archive/2021/10/new-puritans-mob-justice-canceled/619818/.
Accessed April 19, 2022.

Archer, S. L. "Five Failings of the Great Barrington Declaration's Dangerous Plan for
COVID-19 Natural Herd Immunity." *Conversation*, November 2, 2020. https://thecon
versation.com/5-failings-of-the-great-barrington-declarations-dangerous-plan-for
-covid-19-natural-herd-immunity-148975. Accessed April 19, 2022.

Belluz, J. "The CDC's "Word Ban" May Be Politics as Usual. But It's Still Concerning." *Vox*.
https://www.vox.com/2017/12/18/16792124/cdc-word-ban-science. Updated December 20, 2017. Accessed April 19, 2022.

Davis, N., and J. Glenza. "Why UK Has Been Less Keen Than US to Give Covid Jab to
Children." *Guardian*, December 15, 2021. https://www.theguardian.com/world/2021
/dec/15/why-uk-has-been-less-keen-than-us-to-give-covid-jab-to-children. Accessed
September 12, 2022.

Florko, N. "The CDC Has Always Been an Apolitical Island. That's Left It Defenseless
against Trump." *STAT News*, July 13, 2020. https://www.statnews.com/2020/07/13
/cdc-apolitical-island-defenseless/. Accessed April 19, 2022.

Freeman, J. "Now She Tells Us." *Wall Street Journal*, January 10, 2022. https://www.wsj.com
/articles/now-she-tells-us-11641843802. Accessed April 19, 2022.

"Great Barrington Declaration." Wikipedia. https://en.wikipedia.org/wiki/Great_Barrington
_Declaration. Accessed April 19, 2022.

"Guidance for COVID-19 Prevention in K-12 Schools." Centers for Disease Control and Prevention. https://www.cdc.gov/coronavirus/2019-ncov/community/schools-childcare
/k-12-guidance.html. Updated January 13, 2022. Accessed April 19, 2022.

Gump, B. B. "The Great Barrington Declaration: When Arrogance Leads to Recklessness."
US News and World Report, November 6, 2020. https://www.usnews.com/news
/healthiest-communities/articles/2020-11-06/when-scientists-arrogance-leads-to
-recklessness-the-great-barrington-declaration. Accessed April 19, 2022.

Levine, J. "Powerful Teachers Union Influenced CDC on School Reopenings, Emails
Show." *New York Post*, May 1, 2021. https://nypost.com/2021/05/01/teachers-union
-collaborated-with-cdc-on-school-reopening-emails/. Accessed April 19, 2022.

Madara, J. L. "Speaking Out against Structural Racism at JAMA and Across Health Care."
American Medical Association. https://www.ama-assn.org/about/leadership/speaking
-out-against-structural-racism-jama-and-across-health-care. Published March 10, 2021.
Accessed April 19, 2022.

Orwell, G. "As I Please." *Tribune*, June 9, 1944. http://www.telelib.com/authors/O/Orwell
George/essay/tribune/AsIPlease19440609.html. Accessed April 19, 2022.

O'Toole, G. "I Disapprove of What You Say, but I Will Defend to the Death Your Right to
Say It." Quote Investigator. https://quoteinvestigator.com/2015/06/01/defend-say/.
Accessed April 19, 2022.

Rayner, T. "Meaning Is Use: Wittgenstein on the Limits of Language." *Philosophy for
Change* blog. https://philosophyforchange.wordpress.com/2014/03/11/meaning
-is-use-wittgenstein-on-the-limits-of-language/. Published March 11, 2014. Accessed
April 19, 2022.

Resnick, B. "The Great Barrington Declaration Is an Ethical Nightmare." *Vox*, Octo-
    ber 16, 2020. https://www.vox.com/science-and-health/21517702/great-barrington
    -declaration-john-snow-memorandum-explained-herd-immunity. Accessed
    April 19, 2022.
Schoffstall, J. "CDC Tightened Masking Guidelines after Threats from Teachers Union,
    Emails Show." *Fox News*, September 8, 2021. https://www.foxnews.com/politics/cdc
    -tightened-masking-guidelines-after-threats-from-teachers-union. Accessed April 19,
    2022.
Sun, L. H., and J. Eilperin. "CDC Gets List of Forbidden Words: Fetus, Transgender,
    Diversity." *Washington Post*, December 15, 2017. https://www.washingtonpost.com
    /national/health-science/cdc-gets-list-of-forbidden-words-fetus-transgender-diversity
    /2017/12/15/f503837a-e1cf-11e7-89e8-edec16379010_story.html. Accessed April 19,
    2022.

Foundations

A vision for a liberal public health is inextricable from the founding values of our field. Here are some thoughts on the philosophical structures that underlie public health and how they are strengthened by a liberal approach.

WHAT STORIES WILL WE
TELL ABOUT COVID-19?

This book is not about COVID-19, yet COVID haunts it. As I noted in the introduction, the motivation behind it emerged from my disappointment with the way we were approaching the pandemic on many fronts. So it seems appropriate that I start these essays with one about COVID. As I have wrestled with understanding the disease's impact on the world and on public health, I've found myself reflecting not just on the pandemic but also on its historical and political roots. As I reflected on history, it struck me that no matter what happened in the past—no matter how tumultuous an era, how disruptive a war or a plague, how shocking a sudden turn of events—everything that has ever occurred, the immense variety of historical incident, ultimately becomes the same. Everything becomes a story.

This prompts the question, What story will we tell about COVID? More broadly, How do our stories influence the way we think of a liberal public health agenda? The story of the pandemic was more than just a story of the emergence and behavior of a virus. It was also a story of the social, economic, scientific, and political context in which the virus emerged and of the intersection of these forces within complex, dynamic systems. I realize this makes it difficult to predict which stories will rise to the surface of the overarching narrative of the pandemic, yet it is important for us to try. The stories we tell about health determine whether we engage well with the present moment or whether we fail to do so. The stories we tell also have implications for the broader liberal project we are engaged in. Our societal values are embedded within our stories and conveyed by them; if our stories reflect a positive vision of the liberal order's capacity to progress and improve, they can help sustain momentum toward a better world. If our stories reject the values that underlie such progress, they can shape a context that is hostile to our liberal inheritance.

With this in mind, I will suggest four key narratives that I think have emerged from the broader story of the pandemic and that have the potential to help define the overall COVID narrative in the years to come.

The first narrative defining the COVID moment is that of scientific excellence. The speed with which a COVID vaccine was developed, supported by mRNA technology, reflects a new era in cutting-edge science. This narrative is powerful for two key reasons. The first is that this latest vaccine technology is indeed new and impressive and began the long-awaited process of helping return us to our families, friends, colleagues—to our lives. Second, it is powerful because of how closely it aligns with the way we already tend to think about health. We often consider health in terms of treatment—doctors and medicines—that can cure us when we are sick rather than in terms of the structural forces in society that shape whether we get sick to begin with. We tend to confuse health (the state of not being sick) with health care (what we turn to when sickness strikes), which has led us to invest vast sums in health care at the expense of the core forces that shape health. The success of vaccines demonstrates that this investment is indeed central to supporting scientific excellence, but our story of health, and of COVID, is incomplete if it is confined to science and treatment alone.

The narrative of scientific excellence did not come out of nowhere. The methodologies that generated the advances we have seen are the product of a tradition with roots in the Enlightenment and the Scientific Revolution. These historical periods both informed and were informed by the principles that birthed our present liberal system. When we celebrate science, then, we also celebrate the small-*l* liberal principles that allow scientific reasoning to flourish.

But science alone cannot cure all the ills that generate poor health in society. This leads to the second core narrative of the pandemic, and arguably the central one—the presence of inequities. These include, centrally, inequities in morbidity and mortality, inequities in who bears the burden of the steps we have taken to mitigate the virus, and inequities in vaccine uptake. When COVID struck, it soon became clear that certain groups—such as Black Americans, people over sixty-five, and people with underlying health conditions—were more vulnerable to the virus. These inequities were shaped by marginalizing, social and economic injustice, and other foundational forces in our society. The story of COVID is in large part the story of these forces. That Black Americans were twice as likely to die from COVID as white Americans and that nursing homes and care facilities were uniquely vulnerable to the disease reflect problems that predate the pandemic, pointing to the need to address the roots of these inequities.

These inequities have also come to define who has most strongly felt the consequences of our efforts to mitigate the pandemic. COVID caused us to embrace extraordinary measures, shutting down society and incurring severe economic costs in the process. The pandemic led to significant job losses, which most affected low-income, minority workers. When the economy began to recover, with higher-wage workers bouncing back relatively quickly, lower-wage workers recovered at a far slower rate. The effects of this inequity will likely be with us for some time, shaping the story of the pandemic and the lives of those who lived it.

Just as these inequities helped define the spread of COVID and our efforts to mitigate it, they also defined our efforts to vaccinate the population. At one point during the pandemic, Dr. Tedros Adhanom Ghebreyesus, director general of the World Health Organization, said, "Increasingly, we see a two-track pandemic: many countries still face an extremely dangerous situation, while some of those with the highest vaccination rates are starting to talk about ending restrictions." The divide between these two tracks was deeply shaped by the socioeconomic conditions that determine vaccine access, allowing countries with greater resources to get a vaccine first, while less well-resourced countries wait. These factors also shaped vaccine uptake in the United States, creating the conditions for certain communities—in particular communities of color—to lack access to vaccines despite the disproportionately heavy burden of COVID many of them faced. That we had the technological capacity to end the pandemic but were prevented from doing so by all the ways the world is not yet optimized for health constitutes what is surely a key story of COVID.

Third, the story of COVID would be incomplete without an honest reckoning with the loss of trust in institutions and its consequences for public health. The most prominent example of this loss of trust was the way the inconsistent, often dishonest, words of former president Trump created a lack of trust in guidance coming from the White House throughout the crisis. It is also true that seeming inconsistencies occasionally characterized the efforts of public health, perhaps most clearly in our field's widespread embrace of civic protests in the summer of 2020, in apparent contrast to our guidance on social distancing and masks. This reflects the broader problem of the politicizing of public health and the role this has played in undermining the public's trust in us. There is a case to be made, of course, that addressing the public health crisis of racism justified this temporary suspension of prudence. But it is still possible to see how our actions might have seemed contradictory, creating an impression among the general public that ideology may at times supplant public health's commitment to the data. Given that COVID emerged at a time when trust in institutions was already declining, the story of the pandemic may well be in large part a story of how this trend accelerated, making it harder for anyone to speak with a widely heeded, authoritative voice on matters that are core to health.

It is also true that this mistrust of institutions has helped give rise to disenchantment with many of the liberal norms that played a role in creating these institutions—from the scientific method that underlies our public health and medical establishment to the constitutional principles that support our politics. This should remind us that the consequences of our field's losing the public's trust extend well beyond the work of public health. When the shortcomings of public health lead to a broader distrust of expertise and institutions, it erodes the idea that anybody in a position of authority can be right about anything, creating space for charismatic know-nothings to seize influence and lead society in dangerous directions. It is important, then, to have an open and honest conversation about this loss of trust so that we might address the legitimate reasons for it, expose where it is shaped by exaggerations or misinformation, and construct a story that can honestly speak of a world where our institutions and authority figures can be relied on to tell the truth.

Finally, a core narrative of the pandemic is that, as bad as COVID was, it could have been far worse. COVID was a disaster. Yet compared with past pandemics, the virus itself was nowhere near as lethal as it might have been. A future pandemic could combine the high transmissibility of COVID with the lethality of, say, SARS, or even the Black Death. While the bubonic plague may seem historically remote, there is no reason we could not see something as deadly strike in our own time. The better we understand this, the more the stories we tell about COVID can support our efforts to build a world that is no longer vulnerable to contagion. This is, of course, where this book fits in. The stories of COVID shaped how we responded to the pandemic and how we will respond to future crises. Such stories will also shape our commitment to a liberal public health. If we tell a story that says our liberal inheritance is too compromised to shape a healthier world, and if this causes us to discard this inheritance in favor of more authoritarian models, we risk undermining the work of public health. As such, the stories we tell about COVID and about our field are core to the broader argument of this book as it grapples with the challenge of supporting a liberal vision for a healthier world.

SOURCES

Armstrong, M. "Sinking Trust in U.S. Institutions." Statista. https://www.statista.com /chart/12620/sinking-trust-in-us-institutions/. Published January 22, 2018. Accessed April 19, 2022.

Long, H., A. Van Dam, A. Fowers, and L. Shapiro. "The Covid 19 Recession Is the Most Unequal in Modern US History." *Washington Post*, September 30, 2020. https://www .washingtonpost.com/graphics/2020/business/coronavirus-recession-equality/. Accessed April 19, 2022.

———. "WHO Warns of 'Two-Track Pandemic' as Cases Decline but Vaccine Inequity Persists." *UN News*. June 7, 2021. https://news.un.org/en/story/2021/06/1093472. Accessed April 19, 2022.

Lu, R., S. Gondi, and A. Martin. "Inequity in Vaccinations Isn't Always about Hesitancy, It's about Access." Association of American Medical Colleges. https://www.aamc.org/news -insights/inequity-vaccinations-isn-t-always-about-hesitancy-it-s-about-access. Published April 12, 2021. Accessed April 19, 2022.

"Nearly One-Third of U.S. Coronavirus Deaths Are Linked to Nursing Homes." *New York Times*. https://www.nytimes.com/interactive/2020/us/coronavirus-nursing-homes .html. Updated June 1, 2021. Accessed April 19, 2022.

Neuman, S. "COVID-19 Death Rate for Black Americans Twice That for Whites, New Report Says." *NPR*, August 13, 2020. https://www.npr.org/sections/coronavirus-live -updates/2020/08/13/902261618/covid-19-death-rate-for-black-americans-twice-that -for-whites-new-report-says. Accessed April 19, 2022.

LIBERTY AND HEALTH?

On September 11, 2001, I was in New York City. As I remember the event and its aftermath, I recall the palpable fear in the city. In the days after the 9/11 attacks, I started to see this fear reflected at the national political level, among lawmakers and eventually in the laws they passed. The Patriot Act, passed with near-unanimous support in the Senate, emerged from this climate of fear.

Much about the Patriot Act has since been rethought. It has been seen as at best an overreach and at worst constitutionally dubious, leading to no-fly lists and the discriminatory targeting of Muslims. Given how controversial it has become, it is important to remember how reasonable the act seemed at the time it was passed; how, gripped as we were by fear, we were able to see its broad provisions for pursuing terrorists as a rational response to the threat we seemed to face. What many have since regarded as illiberal overreach looked, in the context of fear, like prudent policymaking. This is worth noting as we consider the habits of mind that lead to illiberal thinking. Small-*l* liberalism emerged from an intellectual culture that prized reason above all else. During the Enlightenment, thinkers tried to pursue lines of inquiry based on empiricism rather than on the passions of the moment. Illiberalism, in a sense, reflects the opposite of this, often emerging from climates of collective stress or fear. Such feelings can persuade us to put aside reason and embrace some illiberalism to make us feel safer in a dangerous world. Maintaining a liberal public health means recognizing when we are making choices in this state of mind and working, in such moments, to keep reason always in view.

Nearly two decades after September 11, 2001, March 2020 put us in a similar state of fear with the emergence of a novel pathogen that would eventually kill roughly as many Americans each day as we lost on 9/11. As the new coronavirus swept the world, the fear of it was amplified across a range of media. Headlines from that time reflect how quickly we came to see the virus as a threat:

"Experts Worry about Pandemic as Coronavirus Numbers Increase: Report" in *Fox News* on February 3, 2020.
"Coronavirus Spreads Outside China as Officials' Worries Mount" in the *Wall Street Journal* on February 24, 2020.
"C.D.C. Officials Warn of Coronavirus Outbreaks in the U.S." in the *New York Times* on February 25, 2020.

These concerns led us to take drastic actions to protect ourselves and to help flatten the epidemic's curve so the virus would not overwhelm our health systems. We embraced a widespread lockdown, effectively closing large segments of society in response to what we had come to realize was a looming global pandemic. Like the passage of the Patriot Act, this dramatic action seemed a reasonable response given the threat we appeared to face and our information at the time. In hindsight it remains a sensible choice in the context of the moment when we made it.

But that context soon changed. As we entered the summer of 2020 with the lockdowns largely still in place, we began to have conversations weighing their public health utility against their economic consequences (consequences that were themselves deeply significant for health). These conversations also included the issue of keeping schools closed, with the threat of the virus on one hand and the long-term health consequences of disrupting students' education on the other.

As with any honest conversation about health, these discussions involved difficult trade-offs. They represented an effort to find the "least worst" options in a time of unprecedented danger. Such conversations would be hard enough in a context of civility and mutual respect, and this was not the context in which they unfolded during COVID-19. It did not take long for these discussions to become politicized, vehemently so, with favoring lockdowns and mask wearing viewed as a left-wing position and opposing such measures identified with conservatives. Informing— indeed, inflaming—all of this were the words and actions of former president Trump. The White House's messaging on the virus changed constantly, sometimes even minute by minute, as the president leaned into his strategy of governing by tweet. Trump's tendency to weigh in on everything, to undercut the advice of experts, and to project a cavalier approach to COVID even when he himself caught the virus helped ensure that the conversation about the hard choices necessary to address the pandemic would remain dysfunctional.

It is important to note that, while this conversation may have seemed superficially to be about civil liberties—how much constraint we are willing to accept in the name of health—this was not really what was happening. The public conversation was soon hijacked by simplistic reductions ("Masks are good!" "No, masks are bad!") that left no room for the important, nuanced conversations we should have been having. Because—let's face it—masks are a minor imposition. Steps like closing schools or shutting down the economy, on the other hand, are not minor. So long as we confuse the superficial with the substantive, we will find it difficult, if not impossible, to have the honest, adult conversations about health that can move us forward in a crisis. Such conversations are necessary for maintaining the reasoned context that supports a liberal response to problems rather than a draconian approach based on fear. And they are necessary for balancing the trade-offs inherent in the choices we make about health policy, some of which we struggled with during the pandemic.

Addressing the relation between liberty and health means also addressing the notions of freedom that are central to a liberal society. Core to small-*l* liberalism is a defense of freedom, toward maximizing human potential and guarding against the totalitarianism that can undermine societies and individual lives. Shaping a liberal vision for liberal public health, then, means speaking honestly about the trade-offs we face in trying to promote health, and about what they mean for the freedoms we enjoy.

This conversation can be particularly fraught in the American context. During COVID, the actions of many Americans seemed to reflect the words attributed to Patrick Henry, "Give me liberty or give me death!" In shunning masks and physical distancing and arguing against lockdowns, some Americans were acting from the mistaken belief that the pandemic was a hoax, or at least overblown. But many did indeed seem well aware of the risks and nevertheless preferred to live in proximity to peril rather than accept anything that seemed to constrain liberty, even the not very onerous step of wearing a mask.

It is true that shaping a healthier world can sometimes mean the trade-off of accepting certain constraints. But we accept these trade-offs all the time. Imagine, for example, a group of people all meeting for a rally against masks and lockdowns. After it's over, when they return to their cars to drive home, the vast majority will accept the slight constraint on individual liberty that comes with wearing a seat belt for the ride. This reflects the willingness among many, even those ostensibly most opposed to constraints on individual liberty, to accept such constraints when they serve the interest of health and safety. Seen in this light, the choice to become upset about them can seem arbitrary and politically motivated rather than shaped by any reasoned consideration.

Yet it is important to remember that public health itself can struggle with these trade-offs, becoming just as stubborn about the need to impose lockdowns as many were about resisting them. The consequence of this is that nobody ends up doing what is best for health—public health becomes dogmatic in its embrace of lockdowns without concern for their socioeconomic costs, and the public becomes reflexive in dismissing any public health guidance no matter how reasonable or data informed it may be.

It is worth, then, returning to motivations. Are we acting based on fear? Or are our priorities guided by reason? These questions can help us weigh the trade-offs between liberty and health and make sure that, when we do decide that some degree of freedom must be curtailed, we carry out this choice in a way that is data informed, democratically accountable, liberal.

So what does all this mean? It means that we should indeed be having a robust conversation about the intersection of liberty and health, but that this conversation should always be informed by core values, by a desire to shape a world where we are truly free because we are truly healthy, and by a reasoned understanding of the trade-offs involved in shaping such a world. It is a valid consideration, always, to think about how much we are willing to do for health, how much economic pain we are willing to endure for the feeling of short-term security. This entails difficult choices, a willingness to be honest with ourselves about the data, and a less zero-sum understanding of freedom. Patrick Henry was wrong: the choice is not between liberty and death. There is a middle ground, supporting both liberty and health, and it is there for us to claim if only we are wise enough to see it. Striking this balance reflects the reasoned moderation that defines the liberal project. A liberal public health is one that weighs pragmatism and necessity, working always based on data rather than on fear. The next chapter will take a deeper look at how fear can shape our decision-making and cause us to make choices that are not always in the best interests of health.

SOURCES

Aaro, D. "Experts Worry about Pandemic as Coronavirus Numbers Increase: Report."
  Fox News, February 3, 2020. https://www.foxnews.com/health/experts-worry-about
  -pandemic-coronavirus-numbers-increase. Accessed April 20, 2022.

Andrews, E. "Patrick Henry's 'Liberty or Death' Speech." History.com. https://www.history
  .com/news/patrick-henrys-liberty-or-death-speech-240-years-ago. Published March 22,
  2015. Updated August 22, 2018. Accessed April 20, 2022.

Belluck, P., and N. Weiland. "C.D.C. Officials Warn of Coronavirus Outbreaks in the U.S."
  New York Times, February 25, 2020. https://www.nytimes.com/2020/02/25/health
  /coronavirus-us.html. Updated March 9, 2020. Accessed April 20, 2022.

Haroun, A. "Daily COVID-19 Death Toll in the US Passes 3,000—More Than the Death Toll
  from the 9/11 Tragedy." *Business Insider*, December 9, 2020. https://www.businessin
  sider.com/daily-us-covid-19-deaths-higher-than-911-death-toll-2020-12. Accessed
  April 20, 2022.

Purnell, N. "Coronavirus Spreads Outside China as Officials' Worries Mount." *Wall Street
  Journal*. https://www.wsj.com/articles/coronavirus-spreads-outside-china-as-officials
  -worries-mount-11582473370. Updated February 24, 2020. Accessed April 20, 2022.

"Surveillance under the USA/Patriot Act." American Civil Liberties Union. https://www
  .aclu.org/other/surveillance-under-usapatriot-act. Accessed April 20, 2022.

"USA PATRIOT Act: Preserving Life and Liberty." US Department of Justice. https://www
  .justice.gov/archive/ll/highlights.htm. Accessed April 20, 2022.

FEAR

During COVID-19, I found myself thinking a fair bit about fears. As dean of a school of public health, I often found myself managing both my own fear about the evolving pandemic and the fear of members of our community, balancing what the data suggested we might do with what we were afraid of. Fundamentally I have been asking myself, What role does fear play in our decision-making? How do we reckon with its influence? As I discussed in the previous chapter, fear has the power to overwhelm the reason that sustains a liberal framework. Given that fear can be a driver of illiberalism, let's take a moment to think about fear, to better understand it, as a move toward minimizing its sway in our lives and in public health.

I will begin with some numbers. If you live in the United States, your odds of being killed by a foreign-born terrorist on American soil are one in 3.64 million. This places risk of death from terrorism far below risk from other causes of death, such as, for example, drowning, which is fifth among leading causes of unintentional injury and death in the United States. Yet drowning risk has not shaped our politics and society for decades, motivated sweeping legislation like the Patriot Act, nor has it helped justify an annual defense budget of roughly $700 billion. This is arguably because drowning, while more widespread, does not receive the same publicity as terror attacks, allowing terrorism to generate a fear disproportionate to the risk it poses.

The role of fear in shaping our response to threats was deeply relevant to the COVID moment. This fear is understandable. COVID was a catastrophe. First there were the initial rumblings of trouble thousands of miles away. Next came the growing awareness that the virus was no minor concern, that it had the makings of a global threat. Finally there were the signs of the pandemic's inexorable spread, including devastation in Italy, the digging of huge burial pits in Iran, and the first reported case in the United States.

In the face of this, fear motivated us to dramatically change how we live our lives. We may prefer to think we made these changes because we were following the science of the pandemic and adhering to government policies curtailing our actions in the name of health. And to some extent we were. But as we in public health well know, top-down interventions can do only so much. During the pandemic, compliance with public health measures was motivated by a range of factors, not least of which was fear. A National Bureau of Economic Research working paper found that the economic decline of 2020 was due far more to people's voluntarily staying home and altering their consumption habits than it was to government restrictions. The study found that while overall consumer traffic fell by 60 percent, legal restrictions accounted for just 7 percent of the decline. According to the research, "Individual choices were far more important and seem tied to fears of infection. Traffic started dropping before the legal orders were in place; was highly tied to the number of COVID deaths in the county; and showed a clear shift by consumers away from larger/busier stores toward smaller/less busy ones in the same industry."

Much of this fear stems from the way we perceive risk. There are ample data on how the perception of risk shapes our choices. Consider: a 2016 study found that visualizing risk consequences of decisions can generate negative affect linked with feelings of stress; these feelings can, in turn, generate higher perceived risk. The study's authors noted that this further supports a model of decision-making that places significant emphasis on the role of feelings as a counterweight to rational analysis—more than a counterweight even; data suggest it is often our feelings that, in fact, drive our choices.

Given this reality, it makes sense that we react disproportionately to emotional stimuli. So when COVID arrived, it led to many choices that arguably were guided more by fear than by reason. Take, for example, the decision of some school districts to cancel outdoor sports. From the perspective of reason, this made little sense. The virus is significantly less likely to be transmitted outdoors. What is risky is denying young people the chance to socialize in person, particularly during the crucial early years of their development. When the tenuous risk of viral spread during sports is compared with the near certainty of poor mental health outcomes caused by isolation, the choice that pure reason would select is clear. But we were not guided by reason. We were afraid. This kept the prospect of people's gathering together in any circumstances during the pandemic a frightening one for many.

Given the overwhelming role of emotion in risk calculations, it is unlikely we can ever completely separate our fears from our decisions. What we can do is ask, What is the right level of response to risk? When have our policies been disproportionately driven by fear? Taking into account the power of fear, it is all the more important that policymakers apply reason over emotion, helping to lead the public in a measured approach to crisis. Giving in to fear, and basing policy on it, is not as costless as it can seem. For example, in the United States we have long seen a vocal minority express skepticism of the efficacy of vaccines. A key task for public health is to counter these voices. This was particularly true when robust vaccine uptake emerged as key to ending the pandemic. However, if we caution against reopening society even after vaccination has become widespread, aren't we implying that vaccines are less effective then we have always claimed they are? We would not deliberately spread such a message, of course. But perception is reality, as the saying goes, and this is the perception we risk promoting when our actions are motivated by fear. I would argue that fear was indeed the motivating factor behind many of our recommendations in the later days of the pandemic. With vaccines, treatments, and milder variants dramatically decreasing the virus's threat to the population, many in public health continued recommending lockdowns and heavy-handed measures despite the economic risks they posed. Not only was this approach unmoored from the data, it also projected, at times, the appearance of an illiberal public health exercising power for its own sake. This reflects how making choices based on fear, even when doing so seems simply to reflect an abundance of caution, can undermine public health's effectiveness or even harm the populations we serve.

This was perhaps most clearly reflected by our approach to schools during the pandemic. Throughout the pandemic, the data were clear that schools were not hubs of transmission, and that the virus itself posed little risk to children. As of January 2022, over the first two years of COVID, the total number of COVID deaths in the United States among those ages zero to eighteen was about 900. By contrast, about 2,600 children under age nineteen die annually from homicide. To be clear, each of these deaths was a tragedy, and it is important not to minimize the suffering they reflect. But compared with other age groups, COVID risk among children was very small. It certainly was not enough to justify keeping kids home from school for two years and dramatically curtailing their social interactions—which can have deep developmental consequences for children. Yet this approach was exactly what many in public health advocated, despite clear data on the low risk of COVID and the high risk of harm caused by these policies. That these measures were imposed in many cases against the wishes of parents who saw what lockdowns were doing to their kids only sharpens the picture that emerged during the pandemic of an illiberal public health operating from a place of fear rather than from thoughtful, data-informed pragmatism.

Given public health's missteps in the context of crisis, it is clear that fear played a role in causing us to forget our liberal roots. This is notable, since it was precisely the Enlightenment era that helped society navigate the fears that emerge from a lack of reason. During the Enlightenment, science helped show a way through fear by helping us better understand the unknown. When fear causes us to turn away from this understanding, we also turn away from the basic first principles of our work.

Are there steps we can take to appropriately mitigate fear? First of all we need to be alert to its influence so that it does not govern our actions at the expense of the measures necessary to support health. It's all right to be afraid. It's wise to balance risks and trade-offs. It is not all right to let fear completely make decisions for us or for us to play on the fears of others for the sake of expediency. This means basing our conversation about health, as much as possible, on reason, maintaining a sense of proportion about the issues we face. Emotion may always play a role in our decisions, but it need not be the emotion of fear. Instead, we might embrace compassion as a counterpoint to reason, in the hope that this informs the wisdom—on the part of both leaders and the wider public—to act in ways that support a healthier world. It is also important to embrace the virtue of courage. Courage, crucially, is not the absence of fear, but the ability to keep fear in perspective and function despite it. A liberal public health is a courageous public health. We are all human; we will always face fear. If we have courage we can be effective, even amid fear, in pursuing reason-based solutions.

SOURCES

Bulfone, T. C., M. Malekinejad, G. Rutherford, and N. Razani, "Outdoor Transmission of SARS-CoV-2 and Other Respiratory Viruses: A Systematic Review." *Journal of Infectious Diseases* 223 (2021): 550–61.

Burt, C. "School Districts in These 10 States Have Canceled Fall Sports." *District Administration*, August 7, 2020. https://districtadministration.com/school-districts-in-these-10-states-have-canceled-fall-sports/. Accessed April 22, 2022.

Camp, J. Decisions Are Largely Emotional, Not Logical. Big Think. https://bigthink.com/personal-growth/decisions-are-emotional-not-logical-the-neuroscience-behind-decision-making/. Published June 11, 2012. Accessed April 22, 2022.

Cunningham, E., and D. Bennett. "Coronavirus Burial Pits So Vast They're Visible from Space." *Washington Post*, March 12, 2020. https://www.washingtonpost.com/graphics /2020/world/iran-coronavirus-outbreak-graves/. Accessed April 20, 2022.

"Drowning Facts." Centers for Disease Control and Prevention. https://www.cdc.gov /drowning/facts/index.html. Accessed April 20, 2022.

Duffin, E. U.S. Military Spending from 2000 to 2020." Statista. https://www.statista.com /statistics/272473/us-military-spending-from-2000-to-2012/. Published November 10, 2021. Accessed April 20, 2022.

Galea, S. "Decision-Making in an Age of Covid and Social Media." *Healthiest Goldfish* (blog), February 20, 2021, https://sandrogalea.substack.com/p/decision-making-in-an-age-of -covid. Accessed April 22, 2022.

Goolsbee, A., and C. Syverson, "Fear, Lockdown, and Diversion: Comparing Drivers of Pandemic Economic Decline 2020." *Journal of Public Economics* 193 (2021): 104311.

Holshue, M. L., et al. "First Case of 2019 Novel Coronavirus in the United States." *New England Journal of Medicine* 382, no. 10 (2020): 929–36.

Horowitz, J., E. Bubola, and E. Povoledo. "Italy, Pandemic's New Epicenter, Has Lessons for the World." *New York Times*, March 21, 2020. https://www.nytimes.com/2020/03/21 /world/europe/italy-coronavirus-center-lessons.html. Accessed April 20, 2022.

Loewenstein, G. F., E. U. Weber, C. K. Hsee, and N. Welch. "Risk as Feelings." *Psychological Bulletin* 127, no. 2 (2001): 267–86.

Nowrasteh, A. "Terrorism and Immigration: A Risk Analysis." *Policy Analysis*, September 13, 2016. https://www.cato.org/sites/cato.org/files/pubs/pdf/pa798_1_1.pdf. Accessed April 20, 2022.

"Provisional COVID-19 Deaths: Focus on Ages 0–18 Years." Centers for Disease Control and Prevention. https://data.cdc.gov/NCHS/Provisional-COVID-19-Deaths-Focus-on -Ages-0-18-Yea/nr4s-juj3. Updated April 20, 2022. Accessed April 22, 2022.

Saliba, E. "You're More Likely to Die Choking Than Be Killed by Foreign Terrorists, Data Show." *NBC News*, February 1, 2017. https://www.nbcnews.com/news/us-news/you -re-more-likely-die-choking-be-killed-foreign-terrorists-n715141. Accessed April 20, 2022.

Sobkow, A., J. Traczyk, and T. Zaleskiewicz. "The Affective Bases of Risk Perception: Negative Feelings and Stress Mediate the Relationship between Mental Imagery and Risk Perception." *Frontiers in Psychology* 7 (2016): 932.

Statista Research Department. "Number of Murder Victims in the United States in 2020, by Age." Statista. https://www.statista.com/statistics/251878/murder-victims-in-the-us-by -age/. Published October 7, 2021. Accessed April 22, 2022.

THE ECONOMICS OF ILLIBERALISM

We often find ourselves tempted toward illiberalism in times of societal crisis. I have already touched on how the election of Donald Trump presented such a crisis for many, causing public health to tilt toward illiberalism as an emergency response to an acute, seemingly existential threat. History provides no shortage of additional examples of societies' giving in to illiberalism in the context of economic disruption, social chaos, war, or other destabilizing influences. It is worth asking, What are the forces that pose such challenges today? Although our current unsettled moment presents several options for answering that question—including political shocks, climate change, and a recent pandemic—in the United States one issue in particular stands out: economic inequality.

Now, in a free society some inequality is inevitable, even healthy. But there comes a point where it becomes destabilizing, particularly when it is enabled by a system that creates extra advantages for those who already have much, allowing the wealthy to entrench their money and accumulate more, while ever-larger segments of society sink, with no lifelines forthcoming. This has been happening in the United States, starting roughly during the Reagan administration, when a push for deregulation took hold at the federal level, resulting in rules that disproportionately benefit big business and the financial sector (or, more accurately, resulting in the dismantling of rules meant to rein in these sectors' excesses) at the expense of middle-class and poor Americans. As a consequence, health has suffered for all but the well-off.

When the pandemic hit, the ongoing problem of inequality, and the intimate, kitchen table challenges of not having enough to get by with, intersected with an unprecedented crisis to deepen the country's pain. Throughout the pandemic, lack of assets was linked with greater risk of dying from COVID-19. This lack also worsened the pandemic's effect on mental health. Our study team found that the prevalence of depression symptoms in the United States rose more than threefold during the pandemic, with individuals who had fewer economic resources facing an even greater burden of depressive symptoms.

This finding reflects the fundamental link between material resources and health. It is easy to forget this link in our conversation about health, which places so much emphasis on doctors and medicines as the primary drivers of whether we get sick or stay well. Yet this is not the right way of thinking about health. Health is shaped far more deeply by socioeconomic context than by the work of doctors and medicines.

This is well illustrated by a brief thought experiment. Imagine a day when you are going to buy medication for a chronic illness. Think about what that day will look like. You wake up in your home or apartment. You shower. You eat breakfast. You get in your car and drive to the drugstore to get your medication. Which of these activities will be most supportive of health? You might say getting the medication. But imagine what your day would be like if you got the medication but took none of the other actions. Imagine you do not wake up in a home because you do not have one, or perhaps you have one but it lacks the reliable water and heating that allow you to shower and to stay warm in winter. Imagine you skip breakfast because you have no food. Imagine you walk to the drugstore (say, three or four miles) because you have no car. You get the medication, but how healthy can you really be if you get it in such a context? Important as the medication is for you, it is clear that if your life unfolds amid such deprivation, you will not be very healthy.

Material resources, then, and the money that provides them, are central to health. This is why, during the COVID moment, more nuanced discussions of the pandemic were just as sensitive to the economic effects of the disease as they were to the viral threat. Anything that deepens material need in the United States is just as detrimental to health as are the diseases that strike.

Economic deprivation, then, is a daily threat to the health of millions of Americans. This alone would be enough to make it destabilizing, but it is not the end of the story. As the economic status quo has undermined the health of those with few resources, it has greatly benefited the well-off, whose health is supported by increasingly entrenched inequality. This has created a country of health haves and have-nots. We often hear this inequality characterized as the gap between the top 1 percent and everyone else. But the real traction is in the widening gap between the top 20 percent of earners and the lower 80 percent. In recent years I was part of a research team that looked at this gap in terms of cardiovascular outcomes.

We found that those in the top 20 percent were far less likely to suffer poor cardiovascular outcomes than those in the bottom 80 percent, and that this disparity is growing. These outcomes are just one reflection of the many ways money, and the conditions of economic inequality, shapes health.

When so many have so little and so few have so much, it is a recipe for unrest. When the deprivation of the have-nots is compounded by poor health, this feeds a sense of desperation that can inform illiberal attitudes and political movements. It is no surprise, then, that the 2016 campaign of Donald Trump—perhaps the most illiberal candidate in US history—drew much support from populations excluded from both material resources and good health. For example, as life expectancy gaps have widened in the United States, counties with voters who did not share in life expectancy gains were likelier to vote for Trump in 2016. The rise of Trump fueled, in turn, the rise of the reaction to Trump, including many of the illiberal tendencies we have seen within public health. During this time we also saw a growing gap between the country's haves and have-nots in the area of culture, as media bubbles kept citizens apart, creating increasingly separate social and intellectual spaces for those who were already separate economically and, often, geographically. This has done much to reinforce the echo chambers we can encounter in public health as the field becomes insulated in a layer of privilege and educational advantage that can cut us off from the populations we serve and from the alternative viewpoints that exist outside our bubble.

Addressing economic inequality, then, should be a double imperative for public health. It is necessary in order to close the gap between health haves and have-nots, and it is necessary for mitigating the illiberalism, on the right and on the left, that can emerge from this gap. This requires a shift in how we think about health and how we make health policy. Our approach to health is largely a matter of emphasis. There is so much that matters for health and so comparatively little energy and political capital devoted to large-scale structural shifts in the foundations of health. Given this reality, it is important to know what matters most for health, what interventions would make the most immediate difference in improving the health of the US population.

So what would make the most difference in countering economic inequality? There is really no question here. The most difference can be made by policies that support getting Americans the material resources they need to be well. To have health, we need to have money, and the resources money buys. Ideally, we do not need to be rich, but we need enough to meet our basic needs and a little extra for the peace of mind that comes with knowing we can cover emergencies. In the short term, however, Americans need enough to make what is for many an impossible situation a little less hard.

There are many visions for what this might mean. Some seek limited economic stimulus, while some, on the far end of the political spectrum, seek a more fundamental restructuring of our economic system. I would argue that we have played the miser too long in the face of crushing collective need. Now is the time for bold policies that address the root causes of economic inequality and the poor health it creates. This means expanding tax credits for those in need; embracing redistributive policies to ensure that the rich remain invested in the common good; raising the minimum wage; and, going further, considering the benefits of a universal basic income, in which citizens receive regular cash assistance with no strings attached. Some may say such policies are unacceptably radical. I say that when inequality has reached the level we now see in the United States, the radical position is accepting the status quo and the prudent, even conservative, option is countering inequality with measures that are up to the task. Doing so serves two important functions. First, and most important, it helps support the material well-being and, by implication, the health of populations in need. Second, it serves the political function of showing that the governing class understands the scope of the problem and is capable of addressing it pragmatically and with compassion. This helps to avoid the appearance of an out-of-touch elite that is so useful to demagogues and those who would traffic in illiberalism. When a population's basic needs are not being met, it makes sense that they might turn away from reason and be vulnerable to darker impulses. It is up to us to create a context where this does not happen, by making sure no one faces that kind of desperation.

SOURCES

Abdalla, S. M., S. Yu, and S. Galea. "Trends in Cardiovascular Disease Prevalence by Income Level in the United States." *JAMA Network Open* 3, no. 9 (2020): e2018150.

Bor, J. "Diverging Life Expectancies and Voting Patterns in the 2016 US Presidential Election." *American Journal of Public Health* 107, no. 10 (2017): 1560–62.

Ettman, C. K., S. M. Abdalla, G. H. Cohen, L. Sampson, P. M. Vivier, and S. Galea. "Prevalence of Depression Symptoms in US Adults before and during the COVID-19 Pandemic." *JAMA Network Open* 3, no. 9 (2020): e2019686.

Lone, N. I., et al. "Influence of Socioeconomic Deprivation on Interventions and Outcomes for Patients Admitted with COVID-19 to Critical Care Units in Scotland: A National Cohort Study." *Lancet Regional Health Europe* 1 (2021): 100005.

HOW TO GET HEALTHIER AND
WEALTHIER DURING A CRISIS

In the previous chapter I discussed how economic inequality is a key driver of the destabilization that can give rise to illiberal thinking. In this chapter I will address an important subset of the broader story of inequality: the inequality of the COVID-19 moment. It is important for us to understand this, given how much the pandemic exacerbated the challenge of illiberalism. COVID concentrated and intensified economic, cultural, and political trends that had been building over the years, particularly in terms of inequality. It is little surprise that this would be the setting in which we would see a rise in illiberal attitudes. If inequality breeds such attitudes in the best of times, the struggle of a pandemic only heightens its capacity to do so. It is a sad fact that there were clear "winners" and "losers" of the pandemic. For some people the pandemic made a precarious situation worse. For others it was a time of doing well, of weathering the initial economic shock and emerging better off than before. This dynamic reflects the deep inequality of our society and demonstrates that our approach to health still does not do enough to address this. We need to understand inequality if we are to prevent it from informing deeper illiberalism in our society and in public health. Looking at it through the lens of the pandemic is a good way to help us do so.

Perhaps counterintuitively, I will not start this discussion of inequality during COVID by talking about the gap between the rich and the poor. I will start with some data about another defining feature of inequality in the United States: education.

A good way of understanding educational inequality is to consider some facts about the US Congress. There are many ways Congress falls short of representing the American population. For example, 22 percent of members of the 116th Congress were racial or ethnic minorities, even though nonwhites make up 39 percent of the country. Women made up approximately 25 percent of Congress, despite being 51 percent of the population. But perhaps the most remarkable identity difference between members of Congress and the country they represent is education. In 2020, only 5 percent of members of the House of Representatives did not have a four-year college degree, compared with 65 percent of Americans.

There are many reasons, some good, for this discrepancy. We may want our elected leaders to be well educated, presuming that education provides wisdom and perspective that have utility in governance. We know that to have a career within a university or in a media organization one must go to college, both to obtain the credentials that get one accepted into the "guild," and simply because in those institutions practically everyone has gone to college, making this a required "badge" for peer-to-peer inclusion. Indeed, this badge is worn by many in public health, helping to enforce the divide that can emerge between our profession and the populations we serve. Education can also act as a passport to the prestige and influence we saw maximized during the pandemic as policymakers deferred to our expertise. This has been a double-edged sword in our work, helping us apply our knowledge to the political process, but also giving us a taste of the influence that can distract us from our core mission.

I am not here to argue whether it is right or wrong for us to structure our society around this perhaps elitist formulation. It does seem to me, however, that there are plenty of arguments for the importance of representing all members of society in important sectors that fundamentally shape how we think and what we do. As it is, the lack of such representation can permit blind spots in the policymaking process that produce unequal outcomes, particularly in times of crisis.

Let's take a recent moment in time. Imagine that we were, as a country, struck by a previously unknown disease, and we had to make choices about how to handle that disease that had a differential effect on persons based on their education. Would we then be confident that a Congress that has essentially no members without a college degree could always make decisions that thoughtfully support the two-thirds of the country that lack one? It would be nice to think that those in a position to determine what gets done would make sure that their particular group was not overly advantaged, that they would work hard to ensure that all were looked after, and that the burden of the disease would not fall disproportionately on those who are not represented at these levels.

Is that what happened? For better or worse we have recently lived through just such a moment—the COVID moment. To what extent did COVID disproportionately affect those without a college degree, who were perhaps not represented when decisions were made—at all levels—about how we handled the virus and the trade-offs we needed to make that influenced our lives?

Data from 2021 gathered by Morning Consult told a story about this that is corroborated by any number of sources. Fundamentally the picture was straightforward—the principal axis on which we saw differentiation of COVID consequences was education. Those with postgraduate degrees reported an *improvement* in mental and physical health, personal finances, job security, pay, personal life, and work/life balance during COVID. Not surprisingly, this coincides with persons with an income of more than $100,000 a year, a status that of course is more concentrated among persons with higher educational levels.

So we went through a year of COVID, and those of us with higher education emerged *better* than we were before the pandemic while everyone else did worse. Is this so surprising? COVID brought an economic downturn that was unparalleled in ninety years, with tens of millions becoming unemployed. But that burden was not borne evenly—far from it. While economic capacity had recovered by October 2020 for those with high wages, for those with low wages it remained about 20 percent below where we started. This was, importantly, in sharp contrast with previous economic downturns. No recent recession resulted in more differentiation between high earners and low earners. And this came at a time when our health was diverging more than ever before on axes of income and education. Our team showed, for example, that the health of those in the richest 20 percent of the US population has substantially diverged from those in the poorest 80 percent over the past twenty years.

So what happened? Well, the pandemic hit, we were afraid, and that fear caused us to bungle testing and early response, leading us to adopt widespread shutdowns as a way of minimizing viral spread. We then continued to bungle our response, and the shutdown efforts affected sectors that were overpopulated by those with lower levels of education and income: retail, service, hospitality, leisure, mining. Meanwhile, those of us with higher educations, and incomes, were able to spend more time working from home, minimizing our commutes, perhaps working a bit less, and spending more time with our families. All this meant that, by and large, those who had much ended the pandemic with even more and those with little ended it with even less.

Was what happened during COVID avoidable? Were indefinite lockdowns the only way we could have addressed the disease? Was it inevitable that such an approach would do so much to exacerbate inequality? Or could these trade-offs have been avoided?

I'm not sure they could have been. Public health is always a matter of choices and trade-offs. A set of unprecedented circumstances resulted in a rapid surge in fear of disease. This unfolded in the context of a health care system that was ill-prepared for a rise in respiratory disease cases that rapidly overwhelmed a vastly underfunded public health establishment, pushing us to take drastic measures that seemed like the only actions we could take. These measures may have seemed not so bad compared with COVID itself, particularly since those in a position to make decisions about pandemic policy tended to be the same segment of the population that was able to ride out the pandemic in relative security, even seeing their finances improve during that time.

This inequality is precisely the kind of societal unfairness that leads people to lose faith in the liberal order that seems—rightly or wrongly—to have brought about the status quo. When some suffer tremendously during a crisis while others not only don't suffer but in some ways end up better off than before, it is little wonder that many start to see illiberalism as an appealing option. We in public health are not immune to this. Addressing inequality is core to our mission. When we see blatant unfairness, when we measure how it is harming the health of so many, it is easy for us to conclude that liberalism has failed to advance progress. This can lead us down some of the blind alleys in which we now find ourselves.

SOURCES

Abdalla, S. M., S. Yu, and S. Galea. "Trends in Cardiovascular Disease Prevalence by Income Level in the United States." *JAMA Network Open* 3, no. 9 (2020): e2018150.

Bialik, K. "For the Fifth Time in a Row, the New Congress Is the Most Racially and Ethnically Diverse Ever." Pew Research Center. https://www.pewresearch.org/fact-tank/2019/02/08/for-the-fifth-time-in-a-row-the-new-congress-is-the-most-racially-and-ethnically-diverse-ever/. Published February 8, 2019. Accessed April 22, 2022.

Chetty, R., J. N. Friedman, N. Hendren, M. Stepner, and the Opportunity Insights Team. "The Economic Impacts of COVID-19: Evidence from a New Public Database Built Using Private Sector Data." https://opportunityinsights.org/wp-content/uploads/2020/05/tracker_paper.pdf. Published May 2020. Accessed April 22, 2022.

Falk, G., P. D. Romerom, I. A. Nicchitta, and E. C. Nyhof. "Unemployment Rates during the COVID-19 Pandemic." Congressional Research Service. https://crsreports.congress.gov/product/pdf/R/R46554. Published August 20, 2021. Accessed April 22, 2022.

Hansen, C. "116th Congress by Party, Race, Gender, and Religion." *US News and World Report*, December 19, 2019. https://www.usnews.com/news/politics/slideshows/116th-congress-by-party-race-gender-and-religion. Accessed April 22, 2022.

Long, H., A. Van Dam, A. Fowers, and L. Shapiro. "The Covid-19 Recession Is the Most
    Unequal in Modern US History." *Washington Post*, September 30, 2020. https://www
    .washingtonpost.com/graphics/2020/business/coronavirus-recession-equality/.
    Accessed April 25, 2022.

Sakal, V. "An Inaugural Inflection Point: Ushering in a New Era of Marketing amid a Polar-
    ized Public." Morning Consult. https://morningconsult.com/2021/01/19/an-inaugural
    -inflection-point-ushering-in-a-new-era-of-marketing-amid-a-polarized-public/. Pub-
    lished January 19, 2021. Accessed April 22, 2022.

Scott, R. E., and D. Cooper. "Almost Two-Thirds of People in the Labor Force Do Not Have
    a College Degree." Economic Policy Institute. https://www.epi.org/publication/almost
    -two-thirds-of-people-in-the-labor-force-do-not-have-a-college-degree/. Published
    March 30, 2016. Accessed April 22, 2022.

Senior, J. "95 Percent of Representatives Have a Degree: Look Where That's Got Us."
    New York Times, December 21, 2020. https://www.nytimes.com/2020/12/21/opinion
    /politicians-college-degrees.html. Accessed April 22, 2022.

DECISION-MAKING IN AN
AGE OF SOCIAL MEDIA

In previous chapters I explained how illiberal thinking is often informed by a distorted perception of risk. A range of factors can affect how we perceive risk, leading us to make choices that disregard reason. On an episode of the *Hidden Brain* podcast, psychologist Paul Slovic, who specializes in the study of judgment and decision processes, put it like this:

> We originally thought that people were analyzing risk doing some form of calculating in their minds about, you know, what the probability of something bad happening would be, and, you know, how . . . serious that would be, and perhaps even multiplying the severity of the outcome by the probability to get some sort of expectation of harm. And as we started to . . . study this, we found out that basically we can do those calculations, but it's certainly easier to rely on our feelings.

In the podcast, host Shankar Vedantam raised the classic example of the film *Jaws*. The film has succeeded in making people fear shark attacks, even though data show that such attacks are very rare: the annual global average of unprovoked shark-related fatalities is four. The movie's effect was so powerful that it continues to scare people away from water to this day. *Jaws* does what every effective film does—it makes us empathize with the characters on the screen, magnifying their fictional experience in our minds, fusing it with our own emotions. It appeals to our feelings. *Jaws* does this so well that it overwhelms our rational understanding of the minuscule probability of shark attacks and induces a fear we cannot easily shake. Growing up on a small Mediterranean island in the 1970s, I well remember the release of *Jaws* and the effect it had on my own swimming—for months thereafter I was terrified of going in the water even though I knew there were no sharks anywhere near Malta.

When our thinking about risk is influenced in this way, it can lead us to reach for anything we think will make us safer. This can make us set aside principles that have long guided our field in favor of whatever we think will get us through the crisis of fear. Given this human tendency, let's take a close look at the factors that inform a context of fear and alarm in our society, exacerbating the habits of mind that can lead to deviations from liberalism. One of the most significant of such factors, I would argue, is the rise of social media.

There's no getting around the fact that the choices we've made in recent years have unfolded in a technological setting that amplifies the very stimuli—the distractions, biases, and emotions—to which our decision-making faculties are most susceptible. Social media platforms are a new and potent influence on how we think and what we do, and their reach is growing. In 2010 there were 517.75 million people on Facebook, 480.55 million on YouTube, and 43.25 million on Twitter. By 2018 these numbers had risen to 2.26 billion on Facebook, 1.90 billion on YouTube, and 329.50 million on Twitter.

In public health we often talk about ubiquitous exposures—how the conditions populations are daily exposed to shape health. In today's world, social media is inarguably a fundamental, ubiquitous exposure, shaping our lives in ways we are only beginning to understand. It is important to note that there are some tremendous positives to the increased role of social media, and nothing I am writing here should be seen as a Luddite rejection of new technology. The new media landscape has broadened the accessibility of ideas and perspectives, helping to democratize the public debate. While this has at times made it easier for misinformation to spread, I believe this democratizing remains a positive influence by letting ever-greater numbers of people engage with the important conversations of our time.

However, social media has also encouraged some of the most counterproductive forms of human engagement, along with habits of mind that have not served us well. It has amplified some of the very conditions that can cause our decision-making to swerve off the road of reason and into a ditch. If, for example, decision-making is shaped by emotion, sometimes at the expense of logic and data, social media generates this emotion in spades. Platforms like Twitter reward content that creates engagement through provocation, argument, and constant raising of the emotional stakes. If choices are swayed by bias, the algorithms behind platforms like YouTube quickly key into what we enjoy, providing an endless stream of content tailored to our political and intellectual tastes. This keeps us clicking but does little to help us see outside our ideological bubbles. If a news article can affect our daily outlook, social media makes sure we are never without the latest from *CNN, Fox, Breitbart, Vox,* the *New York Times,* the *Washington Post,* and such. It then gives us a platform on which to instantly express our views about this content. All this informs—indeed, incentivizes—a kind of thinking that is not good for making effective, rational decisions. Within public health, social media can reinforce unscientific reasoning, groupthink, and cultural distancing from the populations we serve. This reflects the broader challenge of trying to maintain a standard of open-mindedness and critical thinking in an age of social media.

On top of all this, we lived through the experience of a president who governed by tweet, whose presence in our lives inflamed all the worst tendencies of the social media era. Understanding the Trump phenomenon is inseparable from understanding the dynamics of social media, how these emerging platforms influence what we think and say and how we choose. The tendency of public health to embrace illiberal modes of thought and behavior, as discussed throughout this book, in reaction to the Trump years is then, in part, a reaction to the influence of social media in our culture and on our politics.

When we make choices under the influence of emotion, bias, and social media's power to amplify both, we are in a sense not doing so in our right minds. We are doing so in a fog, one that is easy to overlook precisely because it is so ubiquitous. And our current cultural and technological context has ensured that this is the state in which we indeed make most of our decisions. There are no easy solutions to this problem. But the first step is acknowledging the many factors that cloud our judgment when making decisions. Because there is no escaping the influence of these factors, there should be no denying them either. We need to understand that the forces threatening the integrity of our choices are forever tugging at our sleeves (or, better, shouting in our ears) and we should recognize this influence in order to minimize it as far as we can. For decision-making to be effective, it has to rise above the emotions of the moment and try to tune out the social media din.

Doing this takes having the discipline to rigorously guard against our own biases, our own intellectual complacency, and our all-too-human tendency to be swayed by strong emotion, which is enormously difficult. Given how intertwined social media has become with traditional media, the chatter of online platforms quickly becomes the dominant narrative. And it is extraordinarily hard for anyone making decisions not to be influenced by this cacophony. This means, of course, that emotion assumes a place at the table commensurate with that of reason and evidence. Fear becomes as influential in decision-making as data, simply because fear and emotion are more present in decision makers' minds, amplified by social media. Unfortunately I have no solution to this. We could argue for regulation of social media algorithms, as many have done, yet this has the potential to lead to censorship, which presents its own problems for the integrity of the public conversation. My fundamental point is that emotion is so central to the moment that all decisions ultimately have been overly influenced by it.

This influence is reflected in the data. In their study "Emotion and Decision Making," Jennifer Lerner, Ye Li, Piercarlo Valdesolo, and Karim Kassam analyzed thirty-five years of work on emotion and decision-making. They concluded, "Emotions constitute potent, pervasive, predictable, sometimes harmful and sometimes beneficial drivers of decision-making." They also noted that incidental emotions—one's mood on a given day— can serve as a form of bias, and that these emotions can be influenced by a range of in-the-moment factors, from the weather to how positive or negative the news stories one reads are. In one study they analyzed, "Affect, Generalization, and the Perception of Risk," by Eric Johnson and Amos Tversky, participants read news stories designed to shape either a positive or a negative mood, then estimated fatality frequencies for a number of potential causes of death, such as heart disease. The study found participants who read negative stories tended to offer more pessimistic fatality estimates than did participants who read positive stories.

Coming back close to home, it is particularly important for scientists to resist the influence of emotion and social media's tendency to strengthen it. Because science is supported by an empirical framework with a rich history of guiding human inquiry, there is an assumption that scientific conclusions are less subject to the influences that shape a tweet or a newspaper editorial. When these influences do start to shape scientific discourse, and when this influence becomes clear to the wider public, it can be corrosive both to scientific output and to the trust this output has historically engendered. This can erode the foundation of data necessary for making informed, rational decisions about health within a liberal framework. For this reason, when scientists engage on social media, we should take care that we amplify the best of scientific rationality rather than ideology and emotion. In a time when technology has given everyone a voice, it is up to us to use ours to help advance the data-informed clarity that allows us to make the best possible decisions about health.

SOURCES

"Afraid of the Wrong Things." *Hidden Brain* podcast. https://hiddenbrain.org/podcast
  /afraid-of-the-wrong-things/. Accessed April 25, 2022.

Hern, A. "Algorithms on Social Media Need Regulation, Says UK's AI Adviser." *Guardian*,
  February 4, 2020. https://www.theguardian.com/media/2020/feb/04/algorithms-social
  -media-regulation-uk-ai-adviser-facebook. Accessed April 25, 2022.

Johnson, E. J., and A. Tversky. "Affect, Generalization, and the Perception of Risk." *Journal
  of Personality and Social Psychology* 45, no. 1 (1983): 20–31.

Lerner, J. S., Y. Li, P. Valdesolo, and K. S. Kassam. "Emotion and Decision Making." *Annual
  Review of Psychology* 66 (2015): 799–823.

O'Connor, J. Shark Phobia: The Memory of *Jaws* Continues to Scare Swimmers Away from
  the Ocean." *National Post*, March 2, 2013. https://nationalpost.com/news/shark-phobia
  -the-memory-of-jaws-continues-to-scare-swimmers-away-from-the-ocean. Accessed
  April 25, 2022.

Ortiz-Ospina, E. "The Rise of Social Media." Our World in Data. https://ourworldindata
  .org/rise-of-social-media. Published September 18, 2019. Accessed April 25, 2022.

"Paul Slovic." University of Oregon Department of Psychology. https://psychology.uoregon
  .edu/profile/pslovic/. Accessed April 25, 2022.

"Yearly Worldwide Shark Attack Summary." Florida Museum. https://www.floridamuseum
  .ufl.edu/shark-attacks/yearly-worldwide-summary/. Accessed April 25, 2022.

BORDERS IN AN AGE
OF PANDEMICS

In some ways the choice between liberalism and illiberalism is fundamentally a choice between open and closed. Liberalism opens itself to the world, to different points of view, to the possibility of being proved wrong and adjusting one's worldview accordingly. Illiberalism, by contrast, closes itself off to different views, stifles debate, and minimizes dissenting views. With this in mind, it is worth taking a moment to consider public health's engagement with what are often the physical markers delineating closed and open: national borders. Our engagement with borders in many ways reflects our attitudes toward liberalism and, more broadly, national identity and security, particularly during moments of crisis like a pandemic. Some thoughts, then, on borders in the context of public health, liberalism, and our uncertain historical moment.

Readers of this book will recognize several familiar themes in this chapter. One is that the world is not straightforward, so interesting answers are seldom simple. This has never been truer than when it comes to national borders. Borders and migration have long been some of the most fraught terrain in our political debate. The issues elicit strong feelings on all sides—whether one favors maximally exclusive national boundaries or something akin to open borders. The conversation about borders becomes even more complicated in the context of infectious disease outbreaks. At the core of the issue are two contradictory, yet equally true, realities.

First, pandemics expose the fundamental interconnectedness of people's health. Outbreaks will spread without heed to the lines on maps that we call borders. With that in mind, borders can play a role in containing outbreaks. Closing national borders as early and as tightly as possible during an outbreak, combined with aggressive in-country testing and contact tracing, can help to protect populations from emergent worldwide contagion.

The second reality is that borders, by their very nature, represent lines drawn, the demarcation of "us" and "them" that can pave the way for a hardening of nationalistic impulses and an illiberal turn in a country's politics. Measures to restrict travel, even if necessary, can fuel xenophobic attitudes, since a disease originating in a certain region gets conflated with the people living there, and the work of shutting out contagion seems to entail shutting out these populations. This can lead to racism and bigotry, particularly when it is not handled in a politically responsible way. In an increasingly mobile world, border closures can also separate families, friends, colleagues, and the social supports that we know promote health and make for a full life. This is to say nothing of the economic consequences of closures, which may disproportionately affect people with fewer resources.

Within public health, then, we must ask, To what extent does our engagement with borders support illiberalism and an undue closing off to the world, and to what extent might it be helpful, even necessary, in the face of crisis and contagion? Are border closures worth it? When might they be? When might they not be?

A core imperative of public health is to work toward a world without the divides of which borders can be physical and symbolic representations. At the same time, public health's pursuit of this goal should not stop us from acting decisively, particularly at the start of a crisis, when border controls could play a key role in stopping the spread of disease and when time is of the essence. We must take care, of course, to do so within liberal parameters, engaging in open, compassion-informed conversations about this difficult subject. Conversations about how we can mitigate xenophobia and advance a more open world are central to the work of public health—to neglect them would be to abrogate our mission. But if such conversations cause us to lose a week or even a month at the start of an outbreak, when swift border closures can make a key difference—as they did during COVID-19 in places like New Zealand and Taiwan—this, too, would be to neglect our core responsibilities. It is important, therefore, that we balance a liberal engagement with this issue with the capacity to act with speed and decisiveness when the moment warrants it.

The World Health Organization's changing approach to border closures during the COVID pandemic represents a confluence of contradictory good intentions and the conflict between different, equally important, imperatives. The WHO resisted suggesting border closures at the outset of COVID. In early 2020 the WHO director general, informed by the 2005 International Health Regulations, spoke out against border closures, saying, "There is no reason for measures that unnecessarily interfere with international travel and trade." This reflected an understanding that health is more than just the absence of viral threats, that the material resources generated by trade, and the flow of people (including the health care workers so central to mitigating an outbreak) are also core to supporting health at all times, but particularly in moments of crisis. The WHO received substantial criticism for this position and eventually somewhat changed its stance on border closures as the scope of the pandemic became apparent.

What can we learn from this? There are three points that I believe can inform our evolving thinking on the issue, reflecting the array of complexities involved in grappling with the challenges of borders.

First, the context within which we are thinking about borders being open or closed matters quite a bit. During COVID there was the unique factor of President Trump; his long history of xenophobia ensured that when he eventually called for border closures, the issue would immediately become enmeshed in the broader culture war. It was difficult, perhaps impossible, to have a good faith conversation about the necessity of restricting travel into the United States when the person in charge of executing such a policy was so deeply compromised on the issue. This speaks to the importance of having a conversation about borders and immigration that rejects xenophobic rhetoric, in which political leaders take care not to fan the flames of hate. Aside from the moral imperative of this, when the conversation about borders is rendered toxic by bad faith actors who engage irresponsibly with the issue it becomes far more difficult to have a pragmatic discussion about it, with all its ambiguities and trade-offs.

Second, we are living in a time when the very notion of borders is being called into question. There is a growing movement in progressive circles to liberalize borders, with some seeing them as a racist colonial artifact and open borders as reparations for past injustice. This presents a kind of left-wing counterpoint to the bellicose nationalism and xenophobia that can exist on the right. These political arguments—both of which centrally engage with the question of what borders mean—complicate our choices about what borders should do during pandemics. I should note that, in this context, the conversation about borders and their potential necessity is just the sort of discussion we might be inclined to suppress, as we have done with other uncomfortable topics. I'd hope that an honest, nuanced conversation about borders can help us resist this illiberal urge and constructively engage with this issue.

Third, when borders are closed it becomes difficult to know when to reopen them, leading to complications in our broader pandemic response.

Say that early border closures do indeed succeed in saving a country from the worst of an initial outbreak, yet the pandemic rages unchecked in other countries that were not so effective in their response. When should the country in question open its borders and risk letting in the virus? Must it wait until the entire world gets the pandemic under control? Or might an earlier reopening be feasible under the right conditions? The answers to these questions are not obvious. Then there are the unique challenges that can come with success. If a country manages to maintain some level of normalcy amid a global pandemic by shutting its borders, it can be easy for the population to feel it has "beaten" the crisis, which can lead to complacency, backsliding on the very protective measures that support this success, and, perhaps worst of all, less urgency to embrace vaccines, out of a belief that they are less necessary because there are fewer cases.

Given these factors, public health has first and foremost a responsibility to advance a unifying vision of health based on the reality of our connections to each other while at the same time meeting the practical demands of the moment. This means recognizing the utility of borders in containing outbreaks. Failing to advance a unifying vision, failing to reject xenophobia and hate, and countenancing arbitrary, destructive divides creates a setting for poor health that ultimately informs a vulnerability to pandemics. For this reason, border closures should not be used lightly in the interest of supporting health. That is not the same as saying they should be a last resort, because early in a pandemic is when they can be most effective. If not used early and decisively, they can indeed be ineffective and even destructive, serving little purpose but to block the flow of people and supplies and to fuel xenophobic resentment. Even in places where early shutdowns were most effective during COVID—such as Taiwan—diminishing returns set in as the pandemic continued. It is also true that early shutdowns are most effective when they take place in the proper context, one that includes aggressive testing and contact tracing and the presence of political leaders willing to use travel restrictions in a measured way.

A useful historical parallel for this perspective on extraordinary times calling for extraordinary measures comes not from the history of pandemics, but from the American Civil War. During the war, President Lincoln suspended the right of habeas corpus. He did so narrowly, working within a liberal framework, taking pains to avoid overreach, and making it clear that he did what he was doing only in response to an unprecedented national emergency. Seen in isolation, the suspension of so fundamental a right is clearly disharmonious with core constitutional principles (although the

Constitution does provide for suspending the right in cases of "rebellion or invasion"). It is also easy to see how a less responsible leader might have approached such a move in ways that seriously threatened the rule of law in the country. Yet given the emergency of the Civil War and Lincoln's own restraint, a case could be made for its necessity—even for the irresponsibility of failing to take drastic steps in defense of the broader integrity of the Union.

It is likewise true that public health can pursue a world without borders while at the same time allowing ourselves the freedom to act pragmatically when crisis strikes, even when this means making use of something we may wish did not exist—sharply defined national boundaries. This speaks to the importance of being able to weigh trade-offs in our decision-making about the polices that shape health. Our difficulty in engaging with border closures is an example of our broader discomfort with trade-offs during the pandemic. We need to become better at recognizing that sometimes there are no perfect options. That we might keep such a tool as border closures in our armamentarium can seem to contradict our embrace of a world as free of division as we can make it, and perhaps it is. Yet in an imperfect world we need not necessarily fear contradiction, and it is precisely the presence of such tension that suggests our engagement with this issue is based on the complex realities of life rather than on the ideological shibboleths that can so easily become a counterproductive influence on our work.

SOURCES

Erfani, A. "Closing the Border Was an Illegal, Racist Distraction from a Failed Covid-19 Response. Then, It Became Indefinite." National Immigrant Justice Center. https://immigrantjustice.org/staff/blog/closing-border-was-illegal-racist-distraction-failed-covid-19-response-then-it-became. Published June 22, 2020. Accessed April 26, 2022.

Jones, A. "How Did New Zealand Become Covid-19 Free?" *BBC News*, July 10, 2020. https://www.bbc.com/news/world-asia-53274085. Accessed April 26, 2022.

Jones, R. "Europe's Migration Crisis, or Open Borders as Reparations." Verso Books. https://www.versobooks.com/blogs/2900-europe-s-migration-crisis-or-open-borders-as-reparations. Published October 26, 2016. Accessed April 26, 2022.

Lee, E. "Trump's Xenophobia Is an American Tradition—but It Doesn't Have to Be." *Washington Post*, November 26, 2019. https://www.washingtonpost.com/outlook/2019/11/26/trumps-xenophobia-is-an-american-tradition-it-doesnt-have-be/. Accessed April 26, 2022.

Mallapaty, S. "What the Fata Say about Border Closures and COVID Spread." *Nature* 589, no. 7841 (2021): 185.

"President Lincoln Suspends the Writ of Dabeas Corpus during the Civil War." History.com. https://www.history.com/this-day-in-history/president-lincoln-suspends-the-writ-of

-habeas-corpus-during-the-civil-war. Published November 13, 2009. Updated May 24, 2021. Accessed April 26, 2022.

Schlein, L. "WHO Chief Urges Countries Not to Close Borders to Foreigners from China." *Voice of America*, February 3, 2020. https://www.voanews.com/a/science-health_coro navirus-outbreak_who-chief-urges-countries-not-close-borders-foreigners-china /6183628.html. Accessed April 26, 2022.

Tan, Y. Covid-19: "What Went Wrong in Singapore and Taiwan?" *BBC News*, May 20, 2021. https://www.bbc.com/news/world-asia-57153195. Accessed April 26, 2022.

Tigerstrom, B. von, and N. Wilson. "COVID-19 Travel Restrictions and the *International Health Regulations (2005).*" *BMJ Global Health* 5, no. 5 (2020): e002629.

A Timeline of the Trump Administration's Coronavirus Actions. *Al Jazeera*, April 23, 2020. https://www.aljazeera.com/news/2020/4/23/a-timeline-of-the-trump-administrations -coronavirus-actions. Accessed April 26, 2022.

Wang, C., S. Ellis, and Bloomberg. "How Taiwan's COVID Response Became the World's Envy." *Fortune*, October 31, 2020. https://fortune.com/2020/10/31/taiwan-best-covid -response/. Accessed April 26, 2022.

"WHO's Pandemic Response: From Criticism to Nobel?" *Economic Times*, https://economic times.indiatimes.com/news/international/world-news/whos-pandemic-response -from-criticism-to-nobel/articleshow/81443977.cms. Updated March 11, 2021. Accessed April 26, 2022.

UFOS, COVID-19, AND THE RETURN
OF RADICAL UNCERTAINTY

So far we have discussed the foundational forces that have informed the illiberalism of this moment. These forces—which include inequality, economic injustice, and the emergence of new technologies—are also core to shaping health in our world. Together they reflect a historical moment where much is in flux. This has created a collective unease, an uncertainty in which it is easy to lose our bearings and find ourselves adrift. In such times it is human nature to reach for anything we think may steady our metaphorical ship. Illiberalism can look appealing in these moments, as a handhold when reason seems lost at sea. There is plenty of historical precedent for the emergence of autocratic regimes, antithetical to liberal ideas, in times of uncertainty. It is helpful, then, to stop and consider how we can become more comfortable in the midst of uncertainty, so that we no longer find ourselves clinging to illiberalism to navigate such times. I will begin this consideration with a perhaps unexpected subject: UFOs.

In 2021 the *New York Times* ran a story with an extraordinary headline, "U.S. Finds No Evidence of Alien Technology in Flying Objects, but Can't Rule It Out, Either." The story concerned a government report on unidentified aerial phenomena (UAPs), an updated term for what are more commonly referred to as UFOs (unidentified flying objects). The article contained this eye-catching line: "Senior officials briefed on the intelligence conceded that the very ambiguity of the findings meant the government could not definitively rule out theories that the phenomena observed by military pilots might be alien spacecraft."

I realize there is an element of absurdity in bringing up UFOs. Given the stigma around the topic, it was striking to see the subject raised in 2021 by a range of credible figures, from sitting senators to former president Obama. The upshot of the renewed conversation around UAPs/UFOs is the admission, at the highest level of government officials who should know, that navy pilots have been encountering objects in the sky that do not seem to behave like any known technology, and whose origins remain a mystery.

As a consequence of the new conversation about UFOs, with many mainstream media outlets are taking the phenomenon seriously, 43 percent of Americans say they are now more interested in aliens or UFOs.

The UFO story reflects how suddenly new and unexpected issues can emerge to dominate our thinking and underscore the uncertainty of life. Think back to November 2019. Few could have anticipated that for much of the next eighteen months the world would be effectively shut down by a global pandemic. In this sense, both UFOs and COVID-19 expose a bias in our thinking, a bias toward normality, toward routine. This bias shapes our decisions, influencing the way we plan for crises and respond when disaster strikes. In disrupting this bias, our present moment has seen a return of radical uncertainty—a term coined in the book *Radical Uncertainty: Decision-Making Beyond the Numbers,* by John Kay and Mervyn King. Both UFOs and COVID remind us that we live, always, with this uncertainty. It is sometimes possible to forget this. We can live much of our lives assuming that tomorrow will more or less resemble today, as we grow acclimated to the illusion of predictability. We know dramatic shifts can happen, but we tend to think they happen to other people, not to us.

Yet history provides many examples of big shifts that can shake us out of this complacency. Much of my research has focused on how events like wars, terrorist attacks, and natural disasters disrupt the status quo and shape health in the near and long term. This work has often brought to mind just how unexpected these events can seem to affected populations, how radically they upset a sense of the familiar, the predictable. We all know, of course, that disasters strike. But when they strike, they nevertheless seem inexplicable, shattering a status quo that seemed like the norm rather than the exception to the frequently chaotic and violent history of humanity. We must wonder, Did the 6.6 million refugees of the Syrian civil war anticipate the disruption they faced? Did the victims of Hurricane Katrina see the storm coming as a force to be reckoned with in their lives? Likely they did not, just as we do not always make the leap from accepting, in theory, the possibility of radical disruption to thinking it will affect us personally.

Let's look at the COVID moment. We have long known that the world was vulnerable to pandemics, just as we have long known that life on other worlds is distinctly possible, even likely. Nevertheless, COVID, and the sudden seriousness of the UFO topic, both felt like something out of another dimension, far removed from our everyday experience. In this sense they return us to a feeling of radical uncertainty. This feeling characterized much of the human experience before our present era. For many ages, even the most common events could remind us of this uncertainty. For example, when we didn't know where thunder and lightning came from, every storm was like a communication from the gods in whose hands it was widely assumed we all lived. In those days our bias was toward an understanding of the world that made ample room for radical uncertainty—in contrast with our current era, when our bias is much the opposite.

With this bias comes, I would argue, a certain lack of humility about our place in the world, informed by a slight overrating of what we know. Much of our sense of predictability rests on our capacity to understand the world through science. Many of us no longer fear the gods when we hear thunder because science now tells us where thunder comes from. Even during the disruption of COVID, the expectation that we would soon have a vaccine helped temper the shock of the moment. Because of what we knew about making vaccines, we were able to feel we knew something else, something we could not know: the future. This is a mistake that we humans are susceptible to. Science provides us with a basis for understanding that helps mitigate the radical uncertainty of our natural state. All we have learned through science can make it possible to forget that our knowledge remains—indeed, may always remain—meager compared with all we have yet to learn.

Nevertheless, we continue to make decisions about our health as if we knew far more than we actually do, as if the circumstances in which these choices are made were far more settled than they are. Throughout the pandemic, I was struck by how much these assumptions informed the conversation around decisions made by various authorities. COVID was a novel threat, a time of deep uncertainty. Everyone who made decisions did so based on incomplete and changing information. It was a time that emphasized the importance of systems thinking in our approach to problems. Systems thinking is based on the premise that our lives are nested in a context of ever-evolving complexity. In this context, no choice is ever linear in the manner of $1 + 1 = 2$. Complexity means that decision-making must adopt a more multidimensional view, with the understanding that, even then, the presence of complexity means few choices will be entirely good or entirely bad. Contingency and unintended consequences abound, meaning that the best we can do is align our bias with the reality of uncertainty, try to see as much as possible of the big picture, and then make our choices. This is what many leaders had to do during COVID. Yet we constantly acted as if there were clear right or wrong answers and that a choice resulting in a mix of good and bad outcomes, with the bad sometimes outweighing the good, meant the decision maker had ignored the science and acted out of foolishness or malice. This strikes me as profoundly illiberal, reflecting a willingness to disregard a reasoned consideration of the context in which choices were made in favor of reflexive judgments based more on emotion than on science.

An awareness of radical uncertainty helps us to see a more complicated picture. We need not absolve leaders when they have made genuinely poor decisions in order to accept that choices made in a context of uncertainty will always be, to some extent, compromised, limited in scope, and subject to changing circumstances. This does not apply only to decisions made in times of crisis. The emergence of COVID was a reminder that uncertainty is always present. For this reason, a bias toward accepting uncertainty can help us to create a healthier world not only when navigating crises, but also when times are good. Uncertainty calls to mind our shared vulnerability, a vulnerability that persists at all times and in all places. When we see this vulnerability, we can then work within a liberal framework to create a more resilient society, understanding that at any moment this resilience might be tested.

SOURCES

Abbruzzese, J. "Obama on UFO Videos: 'We Don't Know Exactly What They Are.'" *NBC News*, May 18, 2021. https://www.nbcnews.com/science/weird-science/obama-ufo-videos-dont-know-exactly-are-rcna963. Accessed April 25, 2022.

Barnes, J. E., and H. Cooper. "U.S. Finds No Evidence of Alien Technology in Flying Objects, but Can't Rule It Out, Either." *New York Times*, June 3, 2021. https://www.nytimes.com/2021/06/03/us/politics/ufos-sighting-alien-spacecraft-pentagon.html. Updated September 1, 2021. Accessed April 25, 2022.

El-Sayed, A. M., and S. Galea, eds. *Systems Science and Population Health*. New York: Oxford University Press, 2017.

Holpuch, A. "Marco Rubio Urges US to Take UFOs Seriously ahead of Government Report." *Guardian*, May 17, 2021. https://www.theguardian.com/us-news/2021/may/17/ufo-report-marco-rubio-urges-us-take-seriously-uap. Accessed April 25, 2022.

Huber, C., and S. Omer, contribs. "Syrian Refugee Crisis: Facts, FAQs, and How to Help." World Vision. https://www.worldvision.org/refugees-news-stories/syrian-refugee-crisis-facts. Accessed April 25, 2022.

Kay, J., and M. King. *Radical Uncertainty: Decision-Making beyond the Numbers*. New York: W. W. Norton, 2020.

Pedroja, C. "43% of Americans Are More Interested in Aliens after Pentagon UFO Report." *Newsweek*, June 8, 2021. https://www.newsweek.com/43-americans-are-more-interested-aliens-after-pentagon-ufo-report-1598804. Accessed April 25, 2022.

Phenix, D. "Sen. Heinrich Talks about UFOs, Aliens, and Roswell in New Interview."
    Mystery Wire, May 20, 2021. https://www.krqe.com/new-mexico-cw-my50tv/mystery
    -wire/us-senator-talks-about-ufos-aliens-and-roswell-in-new-interview/. Accessed
    April 25, 2022.
"UFOs and Aliens." Piplsay. https://piplsay.com/ufos-and-aliens-how-much-do-you
    -believe-in-them/. Published June 8, 2021. Accessed April 25, 2022.

WHY DO WE TELL THE STORIES WE TELL?

Our liberal inheritance is more than just a collection of norms and procedures passed down through the years. It is a story we tell about ourselves, a narrative about progress, human rights, and the advance of science. Alternatives to this inheritance, including the illiberalism of recent years, represent other stories. At various points throughout history, we have seen illiberal narratives become the dominant stories embraced by a population and realized that this rarely, if ever, leads in a positive direction. It seems helpful, then, to consider why, among this field of potential stories we could embrace, we choose the ones we choose. Why do certain narratives "stick" while others do not? Such a consideration is useful, I think, because it reflects why opinions cohere among groups and identifies the values and habits of thought that underlie the choice to embrace, or not embrace, the narratives that inform health. How we resist illiberalism will depend in large part on the story we tell about the present moment. Some thoughts, then, on why we tell the stories we do.

Narratives are likelier to stick when they meet these three criteria: they seem to match our existing biases; they fulfill an aesthetic need for coherence (i.e., they seem to "connect the dots," reflecting some measure of order in a chaotic world); and—yes—they are told by dominant groups, promoted by those in power, by "winners."

The first point—that we are likelier to believe stories that seem to match our existing biases—is supported by something those of us working in research know well: confirmation bias. This is the tendency to accept information that appears to match one's current beliefs. Given the power of confirmation bias, it's not hard to see how the stories we embrace about the world might be the ones that seem to align best with how we already believe the world to be. If, for example, we think the world is a network of sinister conspiracies, we are likelier to believe theories that incline toward the conspiratorial. If, on the other hand, we generally trust institutions, we are likelier to be open to what authority figures tell us, shaping our sense of narrative.

The second point—that we are likelier to embrace stories that fulfill an aesthetic need for coherence—is supported by the fact that humans are pattern-detecting creatures evolutionarily disposed toward perspectives that help us organize reality so we can better navigate it. Stories, in their very structure, turn otherwise random events into patterns with beginnings, middles, and ends. Stories are more powerful when they apply this framework to our existing biases, reinforcing the pattern of narrative structure with the pattern of our preconceived notions.

During COVID-19 this was reflected by the evolving story about the origins of the virus. For a long time the consensus was that the virus was likely of zoonotic origin. This story helped align the seeming arbitrariness of a pandemic's emerging unexpectedly with an established pattern. Viruses had jumped from bats before; it stood to reason, then, that this story was a plausible explanation of the emergence of COVID. This may be why it took so long for the mainstream to consider an alternative hypothesis— that the virus had leaked from a lab. That possibility does not align so well with the patterns that lend coherence to our thinking about viruses. For this reason the resistance it encountered further suggests the power of stories that support recognizable patterns.

Finally, it is indeed difficult to deny that stories have added power when they are told by dominant groups—by the "winners." This does not necessarily mean the winners of the wars of conquest that have long shaped history. In our own time it is perhaps more likely to mean societal elites— those in positions of power and influence. A key example of this emerged during COVID, as the country's renewed engagement with the issue of race, in the wake of the murder of George Floyd in May 2020, made it clear that the story of race in the United States has long been incomplete, excluding much of the injustice and painful experience faced by communities of color. This status quo was enforced by a narrative that served those in positions of privilege at the expense of those at a historical disadvantage. Our efforts toward changing this narrative have been inextricably linked to our efforts to change this distribution of privilege, suggesting that the stories we tell are shaped by the distribution of social and material resources in our society.

So, understanding that these factors shape the reasons we embrace the stories we do, what are some lessons we can draw from the way they intersected with the COVID moment? I emphasize the COVID moment, as I have throughout the book, because that was when we saw a convergence of the various trends, including an occasional illiberalism, that have informed contemporary public health. Recognizing how we have selected the stories we tell about COVID can help us to see more broadly how an illiberal narrative can take hold within our field and how we might replace it with one that supports a liberal public health.

First, we should be mindful of the biases that so deeply influence the stories we tell. In particular we should take care that these biases do not cause us to embrace a distorted narrative, one that is founded on falsehoods and fear and can exacerbate group pathologies like illiberalism and the hate that informs poor health. We saw this challenge play out during COVID, particularly early in the pandemic, as the geopolitical rivalry between the United States and China predisposed many to blame the Chinese people themselves for the virus. At times this tipped into outright anti-Asian racism, as a consequence of national mistrust and the crude stereotypes that are so often entangled with our collective biases. A healthy world is one where these biases, although perhaps ineradicable from human nature, no longer lead us to embrace narratives that support an unreasonable, divisive response to challenges.

Second, in our instinct to embrace narratives that seem to connect the dots and align with our preexisting worldview, we should take care that we do not accept inaccurate stories simply because they appear to match the political or cultural narrative we identify with. In the early days of the pandemic, for example, a narrative emerged in the media that some blue states, in widely imposing lockdowns, were doing better, while some red states, apparently flouting COVID protocols, were doing poorly. As the pandemic wore on, however, the difference between red states' and blue states' performance became less well defined and more ambiguous. The complexity of state-by-state performance complicated easy partisan narratives about health in a time of pandemic. This suggests that when we are presented with a narrative that seems to connect the dots in a way that matches our existing worldview, we should think critically about it and remain open to changes in the story as events unfold and new information comes in. It is also true that as we embraced certain narratives about the pandemic there were points when alternative narratives were demonized or suppressed because they ran counter to the prevailing view. These included alternative takes on the origin of the virus, the efficacy of cloth masks, the presence of natural immunity among those who caught the virus, and the potential downsides of lockdowns. I realize I am in sensitive territory here, because in addition to good faith explorations of these issues, there was much misinformation spread by dishonest actors, and it is important to counter such voices strongly. Nevertheless, efforts to fight misinformation verged, at times, on a chilling of debate around certain topics that could indeed have used a robust public airing, a suppression that reflects an illiberal tendency in the public conversation. This aligned with the broader trend of the politicizing of public health during COVID. As the field became more partisan, the stories we told became more explicitly tailored to fit political narratives and less influenced by alternative perspectives. We should take care, then, that the narratives we embrace do not crowd out the exploration of heterodox views, being mindful that when suppression does seem to occur, it does no favors for our ability to rally the broader population around what we see as the best course for public health.

Finally, an understanding of how victors/dominant groups often shape the stories we embrace should influence how we engage with groups that lack the privilege that generates this influence. While we did not know, in advance of COVID, that a pandemic would soon strike, we did know that our society was characterized by deep health inequities, which meant that in the event of a large-scale crisis of *any* kind, certain groups would likely suffer most. Yet these inequities were not sufficiently part of the story we tell ourselves about health—a story more often characterized by the promise of medicine than by the socioeconomic inequities that create the poor health that makes medicine necessary. Because our story was incomplete, we did not do enough to address these inequities when we had the chance, leaving some communities vulnerable to COVID.

This failure underlines the importance of the stories we tell about health. The stories we embrace are shaped at least as much by deep cognitive biases as by an impartial recounting of the facts. This makes it all the more necessary that we make the effort to elevate stories that will help us get to a healthier world, one supported by a liberal public health.

SOURCES

Casad, B. J. "Confirmation Bias." *Encyclopaedia Britannica* online. https://www.britannica .com/science/confirmation-bias. Accessed April 26, 2022.

"COVID-19 Wuhan Lab Lleak Hypotheses Are 'Absolutely Legitimate' and 'Plausible,' Expert Says." *CBS News*, June 30, 2021. https://www.cbsnews.com/news/covid-19-wuhan -lab-leak-theory/. Accessed April 26, 2022.

Cyranoski, D. "Bat Cave Solves Mystery of Deadly SARS Virus—and Suggests New Outbreak Could Occur." *Nature* 552, no. 7683 (2017): 15–16.

Mattson, M. P. "Superior Pattern Processing Is the Essence of the Evolved Human Brain." *Frontiers in Neuroscience* 8 (2014): 265.

Ohio State University. "This Is Your Brain Detecting Patterns: It Is Different from Other Kinds of Learning, Study Shows." *ScienceDaily*, May 31, 2018. https://www.sciencedaily.com/releases/2018/05/180531114642.htm. Accessed April 26, 2022.

THE HISTORY OF SOCCER,
THE BUTTERFLY EFFECT,
AND PUBLIC HEALTH

A key criticism of the argument I am making in this book could well be something like this: "Perhaps there are indeed certain illiberal strains within public health. What of it? Illiberalism is simply too small an influence within public health to warrant concern. We should focus on bigger issues."

This criticism is understandable. I can easily see how what I am talking about here could seem like the excesses of a fringe, too small an issue to worry about. Leaving aside whether the issue really is so small, let us assume, for the sake of argument, that it is. The question then becomes, How much power do small actions and minute changes really have to shape the world? In this chapter I will look at this question through the lens of two subjects: the history of soccer and the butterfly effect.

My favorite game by some distance is soccer. A key issue in the soccer world, which has belatedly come to the fore in recent years, is the pay gap between players of women's soccer and men's soccer. As justification for a status quo where women players earn less than men, one often hears that the pay gap simply reflects the fact that women's soccer has consistently smaller audiences than men's soccer. While it is true that the audience for women's soccer is smaller, this raises questions: Did this disparity simply "happen"? Or were there discrete events in the past—choices made—that, over time, led to the present outcome? The answers lie in the history of organized women's soccer, which dates back to the nineteenth century.

In the 1890s there were several women's soccer clubs in England. In the early 1900s some of their matches attracted thousands of spectators. This progression, building in parallel with men's soccer, came to an abrupt halt in 1921, when the Football Association banned women's soccer from the grounds of its clubs, out of a belief that the game was "unsuitable" for women. It was more than forty-five years later, in 1969, that the Women's Football Association was formed.

It's hard to think that this early disinvestment in women's soccer did not play a critical role in shaping public attitudes toward the sport and in constricting the game's reach by limiting women players' access to the resources male players had. It makes sense that men's soccer would have a larger audience today, given that the sport had a decades-long head start on enjoying the resources and institutional backing of the FA. This advantage can to a large extent be traced back to that initial decision to bar women from the FA's clubs, a choice that has had a ripple effect over time, producing a culture where men's soccer remains (though one hopes not forever) the dominant draw. Within the larger network of social, economic, and political choices that shape the world of professional soccer, the FA's twentieth-century response to women's playing the game has become, in the twenty-first century, a factor shaping the present that fans and players now live in.

This dynamic—in which a seemingly small decision ripples over time and within complex circumstances to shape a major outcome—is an example of the butterfly effect. The butterfly effect is a phenomenon in which tiny events, happening within complex systems, can unfold into large-scale changes. The concept is credited to Edward Norton Lorenz, a mathematician and meteorologist, who hypothesized, in the context of chaos theory (a branch of mathematics he helped pioneer), that a butterfly flapping its wings could create a breeze that, unfolding across time and space, might ultimately create a tornado. (It's worth noting that the butterfly effect is also sometimes linked to Ray Bradbury's short story "A Sound of Thunder.") The core of the theory is the idea that, over time, small, even infinitesimal, changes to complex, nonlinear systems can produce significant effects.

The butterfly effect reflects the dynamics of a systems approach to health, in which health outcomes unfolding in populations are seen less as products of a linear equation and more as what they are—emergent properties of complexity, nested in overlapping systems. Within these systems, small changes can lead, over time and as a consequence of complexity, to outcomes of profound significance. This has implications for how we think about health and for how we implement solutions toward a healthier world. It also matters for how we think about the status quo. It challenges our assumptions that certain states of affairs have always been so and are the natural conditions of our world rather than the products of countless discrete variables rippling through time and across systems to shape the present. Once we see this complexity, we can start to imagine how we might better engage with it, toward shaping new outcomes and a new status quo that is more supportive of health.

The takeaways here are twofold. The first is that decisions matter, and that the seeming significance or insignificance of a decision in the moment it is made is not always a good predictor of its influence over time and across complex systems. The flapping of a butterfly's wings on Monday could indeed help create a tornado on Thursday of next week, or it could amount to nothing. We cannot know and should therefore respect the possibility of either outcome. In the same way, illiberal tendencies within public health could amount to little more than a minor influence or they could eventually dominate the field and even take root within the populations we serve, helping to instigate illiberal trends within society at large. When we take illiberal actions—for example, tailoring our recommendations ever so slightly to fit a political narrative rather than the science—we may comfort ourselves with thinking such actions are small, inconsequential. Yet the butterfly effect suggests that these actions can contribute to a sum total of behavior that is ultimately deeply destructive to a vision of a liberal public health.

The second takeaway is that, given the power of small choices, it is clear that the status quo around health is, in fact, malleable and shaped by the choices we make in the context of complexity. This pushes us to test our assumptions about why the world is the way it is and about our power to make it otherwise. Our choices—all of them—have the capacity to shape health for better or for worse, and we often do not know which effect they will have until long after we make them. This should cause us to proceed with humility and a willingness to think about how our choices may shape the status quo around health not just in the moment, but in the years to come, informing our sense of the trade-offs involved in such decisions.

For example, consider the potential long-term effects of COVID-19 school closures on the health and well-being of students in the years ahead. Education, particularly early education, is core to long-term health. The educational disruption caused by the pandemic has the potential to create consequences for population health that may not become apparent for quite a while, but that will likely be deeply significant when they do manifest themselves. We knew this was a possibility when we chose to close schools, but the decision was made that the risk of COVID was greater than the long-term risk of educational disruption. Yet as significant as a decision to close schools was at the time it was made, it is hard not to think its significance may loom even larger in the coming years, as the butterfly effect manifests itself in the health of those most affected by our recent choices.

Given the power of these choices, it falls to us to make sure our decision-making is informed by a respect for their consequences—both short-term and long-term, positive and negative. This can help us remember that even the smallest of choices has the potential to change the world in dramatic ways. This is cause for hope, I think, as we work toward a healthier world and a more liberal public health, reflecting the power we all have to advance the good in each choice we make.

SOURCES

Bradbury, R. "A Sound of Thunder." In *R Is for Rocket*. New York: Doubleday, 1962.

"The Butterfly Effect: Everything You Need to Know about This Powerful Mental Model." FS blog. https://fs.blog/the-butterfly-effect/. Accessed April 26, 2022.

El-Sayed, A. M., and S. Galea, eds. *Systems Science and Population Health*. New York: Oxford University Press, 2017.

Galea, S. "A Good Education—The Best Prevention?" Boston University School of Public Health. https://www.bu.edu/sph/news/articles/2016/a-good-education-the-best -prevention/. Published May 18, 2016. Accessed April 26, 2022.

"The History of Women's Football in England." Football Association. https://www.thefa .com/womens-girls-football/history. Accessed April 26, 2022.

Polumbo, B. "No, It Isn't 'Sexist' That Women's World Cup Teams Don't Get Equal Pay." *Washington Examiner*, June 10, 2019. https://www.washingtonexaminer.com/opinion /no-it-isnt-sexist-that-womens-world-cup-teams-dont-get-equal-pay. Accessed April 26, 2022.

Vernon, J. L. "Understanding the Butterfly Effect." *American Scientist*, May-June 2017. https://www.americanscientist.org/article/understanding-the-butterfly-effect. Accessed April 26, 2022.

THE ONGOING
CHALLENGE OF RACE

Public health has long been concerned with racism: its link to the foundations of American society and the harms it does as a consequence of this
country's fraught racial history. In recent years our engagement with race
has intersected with new national uprisings around the issue, emerging
as a reaction both to the bigotry of President Trump and to the killing
of George Floyd. This engagement has been characterized not just by a
drive to address interpersonal prejudice or civil inequality, but by a deeper
concern for racism's presence in the structures that underlie American
life. This has led to a radical reevaluation of the United States, questioning whether some features of our liberal inheritance are, in fact, simply
masks for white supremacy. At the same time, the emotional character of
the conversation around racism has instigated much debate over what can
and cannot be said about the issue. For these reasons, addressing public
health's engagement with the ongoing challenge of race is inseparable from
the conversation about liberalism in our field and in our country.

I begin with some facts about race in America:

- Asian Americans are by far the highest-earning racial or ethnic group in the
  United States, with a median household income of $94,903, significantly
  higher than the next highest group, white Americans, who have a median
  household income of $74,912.
- Approval of interracial marriage is at a record high in the United States,
  rising from 4 percent in 1958 to 94 percent in 2021.
- Over one million immigrants arrive in the United States each year, many of
  them nonwhite. The top countries of origin are, in order, Mexico, China,
  India, the Philippines, and El Salvador. By 2065 the foreign-born population is projected to reach 78 million.
- In a 2021 *Wall Street Journal* poll, Hispanic voters were evenly split between supporting Joe Biden and Donald Trump in the 2024 election, with
  44 percent supporting Biden and 43 percent supporting Trump. This re-

flects growing indications that Hispanic voters are more culturally conservative, less reflexively supportive of liberal border policies, and less receptive to progressive linguistic norms than many on the left have long assumed.

These data complicate assumptions about race held by many on the progressive left, a political side that, as I have written previously, overlaps quite a bit with public health. There is always a temptation to embrace the easy narrative, and to ignore uncomfortable facts, when discussing race. For a long time, many were invested in denying that race posed any challenge at all to our society. In the 1960s, and before then, those who benefited from the racial status quo could be heard arguing that evils like segregation were, in fact, public goods, serving Black and white Americans alike. The progress we have made since then began with the necessary puncturing of this lie as more Americans declined to deny the truth of life in this country. This embrace of truth allowed the march of justice to advance. Likewise, there are some who today feel that we have made no progress at all, that white supremacy remains the country's defining feature. But if the United States remains white supremacist at its core, why do nonwhite immigrants flock here each year in such numbers rather than going to, say, China? Why do Asian Americans continue to excel by many metrics? How has the shift in attitudes toward interracial marriage been sustained? How do we account for the political behavior of Hispanics?

Even in the words we use to ask these questions we elide certain complexities. "Asian Americans," "Hispanics," "communities of color"—these words are shorthand for groups of people with vastly differing life experiences, hailing from vastly different geographic regions, with an array of individual hopes, dreams, fears, and idiosyncrasies. The shorthand is useful, even necessary, but it will never truly capture this complexity. It can even verge on condescension if we aren't careful to keep front-of-mind that we are fundamentally talking about people, not political abstractions.

When we balance complexity—taking care to neither exaggerate nor minimize the role of racism in shaping present-day outcomes—it becomes clear that race has played a foundational role in this country. The nation's economic and social development was inextricably linked to a system of genocide and exploitation that targeted communities of color. We did not invent slavery, but we practiced it extensively, aided by technologies like the cotton gin and by a westward expansion that kept slavery widespread and lucrative here, ensuring it would remain, right up until its abolition, a cruel fact of life whose legacy still with us.

It is also a fact that, from the moment of this country's founding, there was an impassioned debate around slavery. Indeed, there has never been a time when there have not been people here who have seen injustice for what it is and been willing to do what is necessary to fight it. It is perhaps for this reason that when the slavery question exploded into civil war, the conflict shocked the world with its scale and bloodiness. Americans of every demographic stripe worked during that war to reckon with the country's founding sin, just as they did a century later during the civil rights movement. It is important to bear this in mind so that we might see the historical continuity of our present-day racial reckoning and avoid disrespecting the sacrifice of the dead by acting, as we sometimes do, as if this country has never before mustered the courage to face questions of injustice. In fact, the oppression of marginalized groups has never existed in this country without the presence of many citizens willing to fight for a more just union. This is a paradox that we, as Americans, must keep in view if we are to have an accurate understanding of history, one that supports continued progress.

In 2020 this history collided with the present in the deaths of George Floyd and others at the hands of police and in the subsequent protests responding to these events. These protests, which may have been the largest in US history, were striking for their size, duration, and intensity of feeling, and, it must be said, for their links to destruction of property and other forms of violence. This was the context for a revived conversation around racism, police violence, and the utility of an antiracist approach to engaging with issues of race in this country. While there is much historical continuity between past moments of reckoning around race and what we saw in 2020, it is the rise of an antiracist approach that, I think, marks this moment as distinct. Past civil rights movements have been informed by what could be called a universalist or race-neutral approach to building a better world. This approach is perhaps best summed up by Martin Luther King Jr.'s "I Have a Dream" speech, in which he said, "I have a dream that my four little children will one day live in a nation where they will not be judged by the color of their skin but by the content of their character." This philosophy, informed as it likely was by Dr. King's background as a minister, places at its heart what could be called the individual human soul, with all its contradictions and capacity to choose between right and wrong. For King, a better future was one in which our understanding of one another rests, ultimately, on individual character, whose ultimate uniqueness precedes ideology, class, history, and socioeconomic systems.

In the years since Dr. King articulated his dream, there has been frustration with his approach, notwithstanding the inarguable progress it has helped create. This frustration boiled over in 2020 as millions asked how we could still be seeing atrocities like the killing of George Floyd so many years after the last national reckoning with race. This frustration has helped elevate an antiracist approach to the issue. Whereas a race-neutral approach is concerned with individuals and establishing a baseline of equality in which all are free to pursue better, more moral lives, antiracism is concerned with systems. Within an antiracist framework, any system that generates unequal outcomes between races is a racist system. Any action within such a system is either racist or antiracist, depending on whether it perpetuates or opposes the system generating the unequal outcomes. To remain neutral, then, is a racist act because neutrality is in the interest of an inequitable status quo. I am alluding here to the principles of antiracism as defined by Ibram X. Kendi, who wrote this in his book *How to Be an Antiracist*:

> A racist policy is any measure that produces or sustains racial inequity between racial groups. An antiracist policy is any measure that produces or sustains racial equity between racial groups. By policy, I mean written and unwritten laws, rules, procedures, processes, regulations, and guidelines that govern people. There is no such thing as a nonracist or race-neutral policy. Every policy in every institution in every community in every nation is producing or sustaining either racial inequity or equity between racial groups.

This definition poses a radical challenge to the status quo. There are a range of societal contexts in which inequality emerges, from education to the marketplace to interpersonal relations. An antiracist approach calls on us to accept that there cannot be mitigating factors within these contexts beyond the presence of racism, and that to oppose racism is to transform systems until they no longer generate unequal outcomes. It is clear that such an approach calls for no half-measures in its proposed solutions, which is likely why Dr. Kendi has endorsed an antiracist constitutional amendment that would

> establish and permanently fund the Department of Anti-racism (DOA) comprised of formally trained experts on racism and no political appointees. The DOA would be responsible for preclearing all local, state and

federal public policies to ensure they won't yield racial inequity, monitor those policies, investigate private racist policies when racial inequity surfaces, and monitor public officials for expressions of racist ideas. The DOA would be empowered with disciplinary tools to wield over and against policymakers and public officials who do not voluntarily change their racist policy and ideas.

This proposal has attracted criticism for the potential constitutional questions it could raise and for applying what some have called an illiberal, Orwellian approach to the challenge of racism. But to engage with racism on the terms set by an antiracist approach would require nothing less, and perhaps more, if the problem is to be addressed at the level of systems in a context where neutrality is not possible.

My own inclination is to seek a balance between these approaches to racism while acknowledging the clear philosophical differences between King's aspiration toward a color-blind society and the antiracist insistence on a zero-sum engagement with systems. At core, we are left with what is indeed a binary choice between good and bad—between racism and the courage and compassion that mitigate it—unfolding in a complex, changing world. It seems to me that we can acknowledge complexity and pursue policy solutions that address racism within a small-*l* liberal framework without attacking the framework itself as a function of white supremacy. It is important to be clear about where we stand on this, to make plain that we do not believe the liberal context that has helped generate progress—but also accepts a level of inequity as part of a free society—should be dismantled in the interest of shaping a utopia. In this we should accept the antiracist's insistence on a binary and place ourselves firmly on the side of liberal democracy, for all its flaws, as the best means of fighting racism and the best defense against totalitarian overreach.

In the years since the death of Dr. King we have made much progress. That this progress was necessary at all is, for some, an indictment of our history in its entirety, starting with the year the first enslaved person was brought to these shores. Yet despite this dubious beginning, nonwhite immigrants continue to come to the United States. Couples of all races continue to have their love celebrated by their communities. Communities of color continue to embrace political heterodoxy. This complexity is supported by an idea compromised from the start, fitfully realized, but ever more accessible to ever-greater numbers of people: that all people are created equal, that they are endowed with certain inalienable rights, among which are rights to life, liberty, and the pursuit of happiness. In some ways it is a modest-sounding idea. But it has shown that it can exist within complexity, that it can serve as leaven in the loaf of progress, that it requires no perpetual revolution to exist. Is it enough for America in the twenty-first century? I think so. But the question is unsettled to a degree that is unprecedented in recent memory. This is in large part a consequence of the ongoing challenge of race.

SOURCES

Asmelash, L. "Just 4% of Hispanic or Latino People Prefer the Term 'Latinx,' New Gallup Poll Finds." *CNN*, August 5, 2021. https://www.cnn.com/2021/08/05/us/latinx-gallup -poll-preference-trnd/index.html. Accessed April 26, 2022.

Berry, D. R., and N. D. Parker. "How U.S. Westward Expansion Breathed New Life into Slavery." History.com. https://www.history.com/news/westward-expansion-slavery. Published March 13, 2018. Updated March 15, 2021. Accessed April 26, 2022.

Buchanan, L., Q. Bui, and J. K. Patel. "Black Lives Matter May Be the Largest Movement in U.S. History." *New York Times*, July 3, 2020. https://www.nytimes.com/interactive/2020 /07/03/us/george-floyd-protests-crowd-size.html. Accessed April 26, 2022.

Budiman, A. "Key Findings about U.S. Immigrants." Pew Research Center. https://www .pewresearch.org/fact-tank/2020/08/20/key-findings-about-u-s-immigrants/. Published August 20, 2020. Accessed April 26, 2022.

Declaration of Independence: A Transcription. National Archives. https://www.archives .gov/founding-docs/declaration-transcript. Accessed April 26, 2022.

Eli Whitney's Patent for the Cotton Gin. National Archives. https://www.archives.gov /education/lessons/cotton-gin-patent. Published December 16, 2021. Accessed April 26, 2022.

Galea, S. "Who's Left?" *Healthiest Goldfish* (blog), March 19, 2021. https://sandrogalea .substack.com/p/whos-left. Accessed April 26, 2022.

Hughes, C. "How to Be an Anti-intellectual." *City Journal*, October 27, 2019. https://www .city-journal.org/how-to-be-an-antiracist. Accessed April 26, 2022.

Kendi, I. X. "Ibram X. Kendi Defines What It Means to Be an Antiracist." Penguin Books UK. https://www.penguin.co.uk/articles/2020/june/ibram-x-kendi-definition-of -antiracist.html. Published June 9, 2020. Accessed April 26, 2022.

———. "Pass an Anti-Racist Constitutional Amendment." *Politico*. https://www.politico .com/interactives/2019/how-to-fix-politics-in-america/inequality/pass-an-anti-racist -constitutional-amendment/. Accessed April 26, 2022.

Krieg, G., O. Jimenez, and P. Nickeas. "Minneapolis Rejects Policing Overhaul, CNN Projects." *CNN*, November 3, 2021. https://www.cnn.com/2021/11/02/politics /minneapolis-defund-police-results/index.html. Accessed April 26, 2022.

McCarthy, J. "U.S. Approval of Interracial Marriage at New High of 94%." Gallup. https:// news.gallup.com/poll/354638/approval-interracial-marriage-new-high.aspx. Published September 10, 2021. Accessed April 26, 2022.

"Median Household Income in the United States in 2020, by Race or Ethnic Group." Statista. https://www.statista.com/statistics/233324/median-household-income-in-the-united -states-by-race-or-ethnic-group/. Published October 28, 2021. Accessed April 26, 2022.

"Minnesota Poll Results: Minneapolis Policing and Public Safety Charter Amendment."

StarTribune, September 18, 2021. https://www.startribune.com/minnesota-poll-public-safety-minneapolis-police-crime-charter-amendment-ballot-question/600097989/. Accessed April 26, 2022.

"MLK's 'Content of Character' Quote Inspires Debate." *CBS News*, January 20, 2013. https://www.cbsnews.com/news/mlks-content-of-character-quote-inspires-debate/. Accessed April 26, 2022.

Saad, L. "Black Americans Want Police to Retain Local Presence." Gallup. https://news.gallup.com/poll/316571/black-americans-police-retain-local-presence.aspx. Published August 5, 2020. Accessed April 26, 2022.

Sullivan. A. "A Glimpse at the Intersectional Left's Political Endgame." *Intelligencer–New York Magazine*, November 15, 2019. https://nymag.com/intelligencer/2019/11/andrew-sullivan-the-intersectional-lefts-political-endgame.html. Accessed April 26, 2022.

Texas Hispanic Policy Foundation. "Border Security, Immigration Policies and Abbott and Biden's Handling of the Situation at the Border: A Study of Texas Voters and Texas Hispanic Voters." https://www.txhpf.org/wp-content/uploads/2021/11/txhpf-report-borderpolicies.pdf. Published November 17, 2021. Accessed April 26, 2022.

Yglesias, M. "Trump's Gains with Hispanic Voters Should Prompt Some Progressive Rethinking." *Vox*, November 5, 2020. https://www.vox.com/2020/11/5/21548677/trump-hispanic-vote-latinx. Accessed April 26, 2022.

Zitner, A. "Hispanic Voters Now Evenly Split between Parties, WSJ Poll Finds." *Wall Street Journal*, December 8, 2021. https://www.wsj.com/articles/hispanic-voters-now-evenly-split-between-parties-wsj-poll-finds-11638972769. Accessed April 26, 2022.

NOT IN THE NAME OF
PUBLIC HEALTH

I have spent most of my adult life working in public health. I care about the field, its mission, the values that animate it, and the steps we take to realize our vision of a healthier world. The argument I am making with this book, then, is personal. In making the case that we in public health need to get our house in order, I am talking about a house that I, too, live in.

One phrase frequently overheard in this house is "in the name of public health" or some equivalent like "in the interest of public health." This phrase is often applied to the interventions we promote with an eye toward shaping better health for all. Through the years, we have done much in the name of public health. We promoted hand washing at a time when the practice was still novel and distrusted. We have argued for better sanitation systems and city design to slow the spread of disease in urban spaces. And we have urged greater focus on engaging with the socioeconomic drivers of health as a means of creating a healthier society and preventing disease from taking hold. The range of this work illustrates the breadth of the initiatives we can pursue in the name of public health. Such initiatives can vary in expense, complexity, duration, and the demands they make on the public. Sometimes the "asks" they make are minor, as in the case of hand washing. Sometimes they demand more of the public, of policymakers, and of our collective investment in health.

We have been able to make these asks secure in the knowledge that they are in support of something that, for most people, is worth a high level of effort: health. We all desire health—for ourselves, for our family and friends, and for our communities. Without health we have nothing. So, when we say we are doing something "in the name of public health," there can be few greater motivations. This is why public health has been able to ask so much of the public over the years and generally enjoy a high level of cooperation.

There is, however, one factor this cooperation depends on, without which it is difficult to maintain widespread support for our efforts: trust.

The public must be able to trust that, when we say something is done in the name of health, it really is necessary for supporting the health of populations. They must be able to believe we will not subject them to interventions that are half-baked or that constrain civil liberties any more than is absolutely necessary in a crisis. The public must also be able to believe that when we in public health see individuals or institutions claiming to act on behalf of health when they are in fact doing something authoritarian or otherwise harmful, we, as a field, will say, "No. Not in the name of public health." Our willingness—our responsibility—to say this is inextricable from the liberal roots of our field, in which telling the truth is core to our capacity to work effectively toward a healthier world. When we see public health used as an excuse for abuses, we have a duty to call this what it is, to draw a line between the work of our field and those who would exploit it to harm others.

Do we always do this? It's important that we engage with this question. If we have seen abuses or overreach committed "in the name of public health" and fallen short in our responsibility to say no, this reflects a dysfunction in our field that we must address. A liberal public health is one that does not let its moral authority be co-opted by those seeking to launder actions that harm the health of populations. The question is, Are we such a public health?

The pandemic moment may have helped answer this difficult question. As we look back on COVID-19, we can see a time when much was done by many in the name of public health. Government, the private sector, and public health took actions toward keeping populations safe. Some of these actions were minor, despite the arguably disproportionate pushback they received—I am thinking, particularly, of masking. Others were less easy to take in stride—lockdowns, for example—straining physical and mental well-being. Some countries took a lighter touch with what they did in the name of public health, trying to balance preventing the spread of disease with supporting the full range of other factors that generate health. Others took a stricter approach while still working within the bounds of a liberal system of democratic accountability. Then there were the handful of countries that embraced an approach that was truly authoritarian, working to contain or eliminate the disease by dispensing with any pretense of upholding civil liberties.

Perhaps the most high-profile example of an authoritarian response to COVID was that of China, which leveraged its powers of mass surveillance and political control toward a zero-COVID policy of eliminating all traces of the virus in the country. It was not alone in its draconian approach. Uganda, for example, imposed the world's longest COVID school closure, shuttering schools for nearly two years. This measure caused deep harm to the students who had to endure this disruption. In addition to the many challenges caused by such a sustained gap in in-person learning—the effects of which we are only beginning to understand—the country also saw a rise in teen pregnancy and will likely see a significant rise in the dropout rate, with Uganda's National Planning Authority projecting that 4.5 million young people will probably not return to school. We also saw an authoritarian approach taken in the name of public health in Hungary, where the country's Parliament voted to give Prime Minister Viktor Orbán power to rule by decree indefinitely in response to the crisis.

These examples reflect areas where actions taken in the name of public health clearly overstepped the bounds of what is actually in the interest of the public's health. Reasonable people can disagree with the value of school closures, but a nearly two-year closure that drives up the teen pregnancy rate and causes millions of dropouts is neither reasonable nor liberal. Neither is using the pandemic as an excuse to seize personal political power, as Orbán did, or to lock down, and spy on, citizens with no regard for their civil liberties, as in China. When such actions are taken, it is up to us to speak with one voice and say "Not in the name of public health."

To be fair, this is what many in public health did. But the field was by no means united in its criticism of an authoritarian approach to COVID. For example, many supported indefinite school closures, with little regard for the harm such a strategy would do to students. This position was at odds with the reality of the pandemic, since schools were rarely COVID hot spots and children faced low risk of severe illness and death from the disease. It is also true that, while few in public health would endorse dictators' seizing greater power in the name of public health, if we are honest with ourselves it is hard to deny that there is an element within public health that appreciates the heavy hand of what the political philosopher Thomas Hobbes called "the Leviathan"—the active, powerful, undivided state, working toward its ends with all the authoritarian capacities such a state can wield. This arguably informed public health's increased politicizing during the pandemic, as we partnered with state actors to use the Leviathan in pursuit of our goals—for both good and ill.

It is noteworthy that while Hobbes made the case for the utility of a strong, authoritative state, he also argued that the basis for its power should be a social contract between the government and the governed. He believed the state of nature for humans is so violent and uncertain that it is in our collective best interest to enter into a kind of truce with the Leviathan, accepting its checks on our liberty in the name of stability and safety. Without this social contract, Hobbes's model reflects mere despotism. The work of public health, too, depends on a social contract. It is a contract that frequently goes unspoken, but that is nevertheless central to the effective work of our field. It stipulates that we will not take steps in the name of public health unless the health of the public truly demands them. When our actions align with this contract, we have the moral standing to criticize others who take steps that, in fact, harm populations. When our actions do not align with this contract, when we even tacitly endorse certain actions taken in the name of public health that are authoritarian or illiberal in nature, the contract breaks down and we are left with the powers of the Leviathan, wielded without the public buy-in that keeps us from verging on the authoritarian. I would argue that we neglected this social contract during COVID. In moments when we should have said, "No, not in the name of public health," we said, "Whatever it takes, in the name of public health." This left us morally stranded, without the standing necessary to make a liberal case for an engagement with health founded on a properly functioning social contract.

This speaks to the importance not just of saying "Not in the name of public health" when the moment calls on us to do so, but of embracing a liberal vision of public health so that we can take such stands without risk of hypocrisy. A liberal public health is one that is grounded in the social contract, using its powers to support the public. It is a vision in which authority is tempered by humility, by a willingness to learn and to self-correct. It is a vision we should return to, and we can start by saying to our own illiberal tendencies, "No. Not in the name of public health."

SOURCES

Athumani, H. "After World's Longest COVID School Closure, 6 Ugandan Teens Share Their Dreams." *NPR*, February 19, 2022. https://www.npr.org/sections/goatsandsoda/2022/02/19/1079899358/photos-teen-dreams-and-downers-after-the-worlds-longest-covid-school-closure. Accessed April 26, 2022.

Cortez, M. F., and A. Thomson. "China, Isolated from the World, Is Now the Last Major Country Still Pursuing a 'Zero COVID' Strategy." *Time*, October 6, 2021. https://time.com/6104303/china-zero-covid/. Accessed April 26, 2022.

"Hobbes's Moral and Political Philosophy." *Stanford Encyclopedia of Philosophy*. https://plato.stanford.edu/entries/hobbes-moral/. Published February 12, 2002. Updated April 30, 2018. Accessed April 26, 2022.

Mundasad, S. "Covid: Children's Extremely Low Risk Confirmed by Study." *BBC News*, July 9, 2021. https://www.bbc.com/news/health-57766717. Accessed April 26, 2022.

Oster, E. "Schools Are Not Spreading Covid-19: This New Data Makes the Case." *Washington Post*, November 20, 2020. https://www.washingtonpost.com/opinions/2020/11/20/covid-19-schools-data-reopening-safety/. Accessed April 26, 2022.

Picheta, R., and S. Halasz. "Hungarian Parliament Votes to Let Viktor Orban Rule by Decree in Wake of Coronavirus Pandemic." *CNN*, March 30, 2020. https://www.cnn.com/2020/03/30/europe/hungary-viktor-orban-powers-vote-intl/index.html. Accessed April 26, 2022.

Prasad, V. (@VPrasadMDMPH). "Pre Covid, I Was a Strong Supporter of Public Health Having Broad Legal Authority to Take Action, but PH Broke the Social Contract. PH Mandated 2 Year Olds Wear Masks, but Ran Zero RCTs to Reduce Uncertainty. Pushed Vax Passports, Even After Clear Vax'd Could Transmit." Twitter. https://twitter.com/VPrasadMDMPH/status/1516200303757967362. Published April 18, 2022. Accessed April 26, 2022.

HEALTH AND THE OPPORTUNITY
TO THINK FREELY

As COVID-19 unfolded, there was much appropriate concern about freedom of speech and thought. While the global community grappled with how to best address the virus, health authorities faced the challenge of widespread misinformation, leading to calls to restrict information that could hamper effective health interventions. For example, there was a campaign to pressure Spotify to drop the popular podcaster Joe Rogan amid concerns that he had amplified COVID misinformation. In the United States, the reckoning over race motivated conversations about what could and could not be said on this fraught topic. The culture wars and deepening political divides added emotion and volume to all of this, and the power of technology companies to effectively silence people in the online space—including President Trump, with his removal from Twitter—significantly raised the stakes of the debate over what we could say and have amplified by the media that dominated the public conversation. It was against a backdrop of increasingly censorious norms that COVID unfolded.

This was particularly troubling because our capacity to contain COVID depended on the strength of our thinking, a strength sustained by the ability to test ideas, to propose sometimes erroneous notions, and to have those ideas improved by the to and fro of rigorous public conversation. This situation suggests that the existence of free and open debate is a necessary precondition for operating within a liberal climate of ideas and underscores the centrality of freedom of speech and thought to the work of supporting a healthier world. That this was not the case for much of the COVID public health conversation should be a reason, to my mind, for substantial soul searching. Any conversation about pursuing such a world within a liberal framework must address the link between health and the opportunity to think freely. Here are some reflections, then, on why freedom of thought is essential to generating the ideas that sustain health, and why it is necessary for public health to avoid the temptation of restricting a plurality of ideas and to align itself squarely with a liberal vision of open expression and debate.

I begin on a personal note. I was never really supposed to be able to do what I do for a living. Where I grew up, the notion that one could find gainful employment by having ideas and working to develop them in academia was close to inconceivable. On the island of Malta, when I lived there, there were really just three options for the intellectually ambitious: doctor, lawyer, or priest. I initially chose doctor, but over the decades this role has evolved into a privileged position of being able to work in academic public health, where I get to help shape a conversation about how to build a healthier world. Had my teenage self been able to see into the future and glimpse what I am doing now, he would have been quite surprised.

The longer I do this work, the more I am struck by how extraordinary it is that *anyone* gets to do it, let alone me. I am reminded of Abraham Maslow's hierarchy of needs, with the basics of food and shelter at the bottom and engagement with meaning and ideas somewhere near the top. For much of human history, it has been all most people could do to satisfy foundational needs, to access the material resources necessary to keep body and soul together. That we now have a society that supports the pursuit of ideas as a viable career path is a rare and fairly recent achievement in the grand scheme of history.

At the heart of this opportunity is the ability to think and speak freely—to feel that one can share ideas, agree or disagree, be challenged, but ultimately know that the exchange of ideas will be respected. In a broad sense this is an inheritance of the Enlightenment. As an immigrant, I have long viewed this inheritance through the lens of America, of the unique promise of coming to these shores. This is partly because of my early life in Malta, growing up during the tumultuous regime of Dom Mintoff, where I saw political repression and violent factional conflict firsthand. I remember one incident, in 1979, when supporters of the government burned down the headquarters of the *Times of Malta*. A key promise of America is that it is a place where such an event could not happen, where freedom of thought and expression is valued and protected. What I did not expect on arriving in the United States, however, was that everybody seemed to have an individual definition of freedom. I have always been drawn to the definition offered by the Polish revolutionary Rosa Luxemburg. According to her, "Freedom is always and exclusively freedom for the one who thinks differently." This, I think, covers most of us. Few could say they have never found themselves in a position of thinking differently—a life without such moments would be empty indeed.

In addition to supporting a rich, meaningful life, this freedom is essential to health. Creating a healthy society is a big task requiring big ideas. Such ideas will necessarily spark disagreements. This is good. We should welcome disagreements and be open to them. This exchange of ideas can develop only in a context of maximal freedom of thought. I believe that of late we have fallen short of supporting such a context. Promoting health requires a robust intellectual climate, sustained by a liberal view of free thought, informed by the liberty to voice ideas, to make mistakes, and to truly innovate. With this in mind, I will suggest three key impediments to creating such a climate, in the hope that by acknowledging them we can reverse course.

First, we have become less able to distinguish between truth and belief. Years ago, Stephen Colbert coined the word "truthiness" to describe something that feels true even when the facts prove otherwise. Colbert introduced the word largely as a joke, yet in recent years it is arguably the pillar of many a worldview. We have seen it on the right, with "alternative facts," and we have seen it on the left with the notion of having a "personal truth" that may or may not always correspond with data. The conflation of what is true with what feels true has muddied the waters of thought. Theories must be testable, subject to change according to the facts. When we conflate the truth with what feels true, we are no longer testing theories, we are expressing personal beliefs. This can make every contradiction seem like an attack, an offense, a violation of our deepest values. It can also lead to a rush to censor when we encounter something that does not align with what we believe to be true. Such a context is not conducive to free thinking.

Second, instead of thinking for ourselves, we have at times outsourced the business of generating our ideas and opinions. We are living in a media environment full of compelling slogans, charismatic speakers, division of outlooks and ideologies, and technologies that deliver all this to us at every minute of the day. It can be difficult, amid this, to sort out which of our opinions we formulated through a process of reason and which we simply absorbed from this cacophony. What is easy, however, is getting swept up in the moment, joining the chorus of prevailing opinion and, when we find ourselves thinking differently, keeping those thoughts to ourselves.

The great irony of this conformity—let's call it what it is—is that the more we borrow thoughts from others, the less likely these thoughts are to reflect what other people have truly concluded for themselves. This speaks to the third impediment to free thinking: preference falsification and the gap between what we might call the performance of ideas and opinions and what people genuinely think. Achieving health relies on a process of persuasion, whereby we cultivate buy-in to a vision of the world that supports health. If we are not honest with each other about what we think, we cannot know where we stand in this process. It is difficult to advance a change in attitudes when we cannot be sure of the true ideological leanings of those we engage with. Nor can we bring people around to our way of thinking when the positions we advance do not reflect our own internal reasoning. It's difficult to convince someone of something we don't fully believe ourselves.

In considering the state of the current public debate, and the restrictions that have been imposed on the range of public expressions of opinions within public health, I therefore feel a sense of loss. It seems the status quo has made it likely we will miss out on truly original ideas, on the perspective of those who think differently. It's hard to imagine easy solutions to this, because the problem reflects such deep technological and cultural shifts. The media feedback loops that have come to characterize so much of the public conversation have made it possible to not even notice that we are in a bubble, to believe we are engaging with all sides of a debate when we are, in fact, engaging within narrow parameters indeed.

The new normal may well be the public health debate carrying on indefinitely in its present form. Yet I must believe that others have also noticed an illiberal shift in the public debate that has posed challenges to our ability to think freely about urgent problems. If so, it is up to us, as individuals, to do what we can to support a conversation that is worthy of the challenges we face. Creating a healthier world will take the very best ideas, and these can emerge only when there is free and open inquiry. In my travels, I have seen what cultures look like when they value such a context, and I have seen what they look like when they do not. It is better by far when we prize the opportunity to inquire freely, to debate, even to occasionally be wrong in public, on our way to being right. Only when we are free to think differently are we free to think at all.

SOURCES

"The Dom Years." *Malta Independent*, August 26, 2012. https://www.independent.com.mt /articles/2012-08-26/leader/the-dom-years-315127/. Accessed April 26, 2022.

Galizia, D. C. "Yesterday was the 35th Anniversary of the Day Labour Party Supporters Burnt Down the *Times of Malta*." *Running Commentary*, October 16, 2014. https://daph necaruanagalizia.com/2014/10/yesterday-was-the-35th-anniversary-of-the-day-labour -party-supporters-burnt-down-the-times-of-malta/. Accessed April 27, 2022.

"A Guide to the 5 Levels of Maslow's Hierarchy of Needs." MasterClass. https://www.mas terclass.com/articles/a-guide-to-the-5-levels-of-maslows-hierarchy-of-needs. Published November 8, 2020. Accessed April 26, 2022.

Luxemburg, R. Quotation by Rosa Luxemburg. Goodreads. https://www.goodreads.com /quotes/6081375-freedom-is-always-and-exclusively-freedom-for-the-one-who. Accessed April 27, 2022.

"Preference Falsification." Wikipedia. https://en.wikipedia.org/wiki/Preference_falsifica tion. Updated March 13, 2022. Accessed April 27, 2022.

Rosman K., B. Sisario, M. Isaac, and A. Satariano. "Spotify Bet Big on Joe Rogan. It Got More Than It Counted On." *New York Times*, February 17, 2022. https://www.nytimes .com/2022/02/17/arts/music/spotify-joe-rogan-misinformation.html. Accessed April 26, 2022.

"'Truthiness': Can Something 'Seem,' without Being, True?" Merriam-Webster. https:// www.merriam-webster.com/words-at-play/truthiness-meaning-word-origin. Accessed April 27, 2022.

THINKING IN GROUPS OR
THINKING FOR OURSELVES:
IN PRAISE OF ICONOCLASM

Americans trust scientists. This may seem surprising to some, given how attitudes toward science were politicized during the COVID-19 pandemic. But the data bear it out—the scientific community has long enjoyed public trust. Data show that 44 percent of US adults say they have a great deal of confidence in the scientific community. This trust has remained fairly stable for decades. Indeed, a core aim of my argument for a liberal public health is maintaining this trust. When it looks as if public health has been unduly influenced by emotion and ideology at the expense of reason, it is harder for the public to believe what we say. Sustaining trust means, frankly, being trustworthy, guided by liberal ideals.

Underlying this trust is the assumption that science will do what it has done ever since it developed its core methodologies: pursue truth through liberal, empirical means, guided by data rather than by other incentives, financial or partisan. It is then worth asking, Do we in the scientific community do this? On one level the answer is obviously yes, we do, though perhaps imperfectly. But what if we modify the question to ask, Do we do this all the time, or at least enough to fully justify the public's trust in us? How often do we think for ourselves, guided principally by data, and how often are our thoughts shaped by other factors? We are susceptible to other factors, though not necessarily in the sense of being unduly partisan or subject to financial incentives. Instead, science has a weakness for groupthink, for being swayed by the consensus simply because it is the consensus. If this is so, then we have a responsibility not just to be on guard against this tendency, but also to maintain a healthy level of iconoclasm, an instinct for pushing against the consensus as a means of testing our assumptions and ensuring that we are indeed thinking for ourselves.

The integrity of the scientific discipline is a key inheritance of the Enlightenment, a period that did much to support an empirical approach to problems. Such integrity, then, is kin to the principles of small-*l* liberalism that also emerged from the period, and that are based in part on empirical

observations about society and human nature. Keeping science "honest"—
rooted in empiricism and as free as possible from groupthink—is therefore
central to supporting the liberalism that informs a healthier world. As I
have written earlier in this book, these Enlightenment principles are the
roots of public health. To forget them is, in a fundamental sense, to forget
ourselves, to the detriment of our work.

In 2015 I wrote a piece for *Fortune* that reflected the danger of groupthink. The impetus for the piece was public health authorities' conflicted
attitude toward the potential adverse consequences of excessive salt intake in the general population. Opinion about sodium intake had roughly
settled into two camps. One camp believed sodium had a largely negative
influence on health, and the other thought the science did not support
such a view. I became fascinated by this, not because it was directly linked
to my area of study, but because I could not quite understand how such
divergent views could coexist, strongly held on either side. Both camps
of the salt debate leaned heavily on their own research, from which they
drew conclusions. On one side there was a body of knowledge that seemed
to support a dim view of salt intake, and on the other there was a body of
knowledge that seemed to contradict this view.

How can there be two schools of thought, supported by separate
data pools, reaching opposite conclusions? When we dug into this we
found that this was indeed possible when two schools of thought effectively sealed themselves within bubbles of unquestioning groupthink,
embracing only lines of inquiry that reinforced the positions they were
most sympathetic to. At some point data on salt ceased being just data to
those who engaged with it and became something else. The data became
narratives—competing narratives, in fact. As scientists began to perceive
a narrative—"salt good" or "salt bad"—they started believing only research
that supported the narrative they embraced. Most consequentially, perhaps, they started to *cite* only research supporting that narrative. This created parallel scientific universes in which conclusions were regarded by
their supporters as close to self-evident, bolstered by what appeared to be
a robust body of evidence. This represents an entrenchment of perspective that has more in common with faith than with the empirical pursuit
of evidence.

This situation teaches us that effective, liberal science should have—in
addition to empirical rigor—a measure of healthy iconoclasm, as a means
of resisting easy narratives and the groupthink that can support them. I
don't mean a cranky iconoclasm that thrives on a reflexive rejection of

consensus for its own sake, but rather an iconoclasm that questions, that asks if what we think we know is as airtight as it may seem.

Such an instinct would serve us well in our efforts to find solutions to the problems that threaten health. Often, groupthink can weaken our efficiency in the face of such problems. A key challenge posed by groupthink is its tendency to give rise to untenable, absolutist positions on issues, which can stand in the way of real-world progress. During COVID, we saw a number of examples of science's taking positions emerging from dug-in, consensus-based thinking that arguably ignored critical nuance. This included, for example, the goal of "zero COVID" (in which success against the virus was defined as nothing less than eliminating all infections and deaths). This goal was impractical from a perspective rooted in pragmatic engagement with the realities of disease mitigation. However, from the perspective of scientific groupthink it made perfect sense. For those of the opinion that COVID could in any meaningful sense be managed—and that the goal of public health should be to eliminate risk rather than mitigate it—no other position would have been acceptable.

The divide within the scientific community over COVID was well captured by the dueling memoranda of the Great Barrington Declaration and the John Snow Memorandum. As I mentioned earlier, the Great Barrington Declaration argued for a "focused protection" approach: safeguarding the vulnerable while minimizing lockdowns and other restrictive measures, with an eye toward preventing the societal harms they can cause. The John Snow Memorandum, drafted in response to the Great Barrington Declaration, argued strongly against such an approach, taking the position that nothing short of "all hands on deck" efforts to contain COVID should be acceptable. These two perspectives became, to many who held them, more than perspectives. They became narratives, and while there was merit in each approach to the pandemic, it became difficult for partisans of either side to see this once they become invested in their preferred story. A call for iconoclasm, then, is a call for being constantly aware of the other camp, so that narrative does not take precedence over data. This doesn't mean we can never conclude that a particular perspective is better than others. But this conclusion should be supported by independence of thought and by habits of mind that steer us away from groupthink and toward whatever the data are telling us about a given issue.

Note that while the intellectual debate between the two COVID camps remained ongoing for some time, the reality of the pandemic itself soon placed its thumb on the scale of the argument, settling the issue in practice long before the intellectual debate subsided. We soon arrived at a place where we worked to safeguard the vulnerable, provided the vaccine to those who wanted it, and embraced a reopening of society. We did this because the evolution of the pandemic necessitated it rather than because of anything we collectively decided. We behaved in accordance with the changing times, even as we continued to debate what was, in spite of our conversations, already largely a fait accompli.

I raise this point because it reflects a key means of escaping groupthink: engagement with reality itself. When we fall into the gravitational pull of a consensus and do not think for ourselves, we are vulnerable to missing the reality of what we are discussing. When this reality asserts itself, it can do much to break a consensus that is not based on practical engagement with the world. We can avoid groupthink, then, through a constant effort to see reality as it is, not filtered through the lens of how it looks to those within our professional circle. This clear-eyed perspective is not easy to maintain; as George Orwell said, "To see what is in front of one's nose needs a constant struggle." He said this regarding the political sphere, but he could just as easily have applied his observation to the scientific community. It may even be *more* applicable there, since we so often consider such clear-eyed thinking a given and perhaps regard a distorted view as more of a problem for less empirically based fields.

I realize that pursuing a healthy level of iconoclasm in science may be more easily recommended than done. It is one matter to think a bit more critically about positions we hold; it is another to pursue a research direction that is outside conventional wisdom about what constitutes a valid line of inquiry. And it is difficult in any context to publicly express thoughts that go against the consensus, particularly when that consensus is supported by one's peers and friends. But when groupthink proliferates, it can cause us to miss important details, ultimately weakening our effectiveness as public health professionals, undermining a liberal vision for public health, and placing lives at risk.

SOURCES

"About the John Snow Memorandum." https://www.johnsnowmemo.com/about.html. Accessed April 27, 2022.

Bayer, R., D. M. Johns, and S. Galea. "A False Aura of Scientific Controversy around Salt?" *Lancet* 388, no. 10056 (2016): 2109.

Bayer, R., D. M. Johns, and S. Galea. "Salt and Public Health: Contested Science and the Challenge of Evidence-Based Decision Making." *Health Affairs (Millwood)* 31, no. 12 (2012): 2738–46.

Funk, C., and B. Kennedy. "Public Confidence in Scientists Has Remained Stable for Decades." Pew Research Center. https://www.pewresearch.org/fact-tank/2020/08/27/public-confidence-in-scientists-has-remained-stable-for-decades/. Published August 27, 2020. Accessed April 27, 2022.

Galea, S. "This Is Why You Can't Always Trust Data." *Fortune*, December 21, 2015. https://fortune.com/2015/12/21/research-bias-data/. Accessed April 27, 2022.

"Great Barrington Declaration." https://gbdeclaration.org. Accessed April 27, 2022.

Orwell, G. "In Front of Your Nose." *Tribune*, March 22, 1946. Orwell Foundation. https://www.orwellfoundation.com/the-orwell-foundation/orwell/essays-and-other-works/in front of your nose/. Accessed April 27, 2022.

Trinquart, L., D. M. Johns, and S. Galea. "Why Do We Think We Know What We Know? A Metaknowledge Analysis of the Salt Controversy." *International Journal of Epidemiology* 45, no. 1 (2016): 251–60.

THE CHALLENGE OF
SLOW-BURNING THREATS

Public health is concerned with the foundational forces that shape health. In practical terms this means keeping our eyes, always, on the long-term, macro-level trends that shape our health by shaping the context of our lives. Because these forces are so large, and their influence runs so deep, they are often best viewed through the lens of history. When we look back and evaluate how historical moments developed over decades or even centuries, it becomes easier to see how foundational forces slowly coalesce into disruptive paradigm shifts. In real time, however, it can be a challenge to keep these forces in view as we balance navigating the changing concerns of the moment with a focus on deeper issues. In a sense this book is an effort to engage with what strikes me as a slow-burning shift of public health's foundations. Our slide toward illiberalism can seem minor in the moment, but when we look at where we are now compared with where we were just five years ago, it takes on greater significance. Illiberalism is a creeping influence, not a sudden takeover, and seeing it clearly means drawing on our capacity to engage with other slow-burning threats. Let's take a moment to consider the challenge of such threats and how our experience of dealing with them can inform how we address other such challenges, including growing illiberalism within our field.

The challenge of slow-burning threats was uniquely illustrated by the emergence of COVID-19. We did not know specifically that a pandemic would strike in 2019. But we were long aware of the likelihood that such a contagion *would* emerge, and we knew it would probably happen relatively soon. Yet when COVID did come, it looked very much as if it caught the world unawares. Our response was a chaos of good ideas and bad ideas, good implementation and bad implementation. Many of these shortcomings can, of course, be ascribed to poor—or at best inconsistent— leadership. US leadership, in particular, was in the midst of immense disruption and transition when the pandemic struck, with the unprecedented figure of Donald Trump in the White House and a presidential election like no other looming in November 2020. It was perhaps unavoidable that these circumstances would shape the coherence of our pandemic response. Indeed, there is a temptation to lay *all* our failings during COVID at the feet of the unique political moment in which it unfolded. This temptation may be particularly acute for those of us in public health, who have an interest—human beings that we are—in not always facing our shortcomings as squarely as we might.

But faced they must be, for they raise the urgent question, If we saw the pandemic coming, why weren't we better prepared for it? Much of our failure to address slow-burning threats stems from our tendency to prioritize the urgent over the important. The distinction between the urgent and the important is something I've previously written about, as have others. The important is what relates to core, long-term priorities. At the collective level, these include addressing slow-burning challenges like pandemics and climate change. Ideally, the important represents a kind of North Star, guiding our broader efforts even as we shift and improvise our way through our day-to-day business. It is that daily business that constitutes the urgent—the activities and issues that emerge suddenly, demanding immediate attention, consuming our waking hours. We have to deal with the urgent while staying mindful that the urgent does not distract us from the important. We must attend to the day-to-day with our eyes nevertheless fixed on the long term.

To use a military analogy, the important and the urgent are like strategy and tactics. Strategy is the broad-stroke planning meant to win a war over an extended period. Tactics are the maneuvers used within the framework of strategy—choices made in an individual battle, for example, or in considering the daily logistical demands of maintaining an army. Likewise, the urgent comprises the real-time details of our lives and work, while the important represents the broader trajectory to which we aspire.

The necessity for long-term thinking that focuses on the important, and the challenge of maintaining this thinking, is well illustrated by one of the most famous psychological studies ever conducted: the Stanford marshmallow experiment. In the study children were given a choice: they could either have one marshmallow immediately or have two marshmallows later. In follow-up research, the children who waited longer for their marshmallows were found to have better life outcomes on a range of indicators. The experiment reflects something fundamental about why we can sometimes give the urgent over priority over the important, even when we know doing so harms us in the long run—or at least fails to maximize our potential. There is an appeal to engaging with the urgent because it offers us instant gratification by being more quickly and comprehensively addressed than the long-term issues that constitute the important. We can attend to the urgent work of the day, finish it, and feel a sense of accomplishment, while the work of a decade or a generation does not produce feelings of quick victory. This is to say nothing of the fact that the urgent is just plain distracting. It is in front of us day in, day out, so it can be difficult to see what is beyond it. Yet, as with the marshmallow test, taking the longer, more patient view is necessary for maximizing outcomes over time, even as we also engage with the daily demands of the urgent.

How, then, can we pay more attention to the important, so that it is not drowned out by the urgent? I suggest we should embrace three key steps.

First, we need a relentless focus on what matters most for health, as a means of keeping our long-term priorities front-of-mind as we navigate the demands of the urgent. In my past writing with colleagues, we identified what matters most as the upstream forces that shape health. These include politics, the environment, our social networks, the places we live, work, and play, and the promotion of social, economic, and racial justice. Notably, each of these forces intersects with the urgent in key ways. Indeed, the urgent invariably reflects the downstream effects of the important, as our daily life is influenced by the larger forces that shape our world. When we see this link, it can become easier to keep the important in mind, as we realize that what may have seemed like distractions are, in fact, daily reminders of the upstream forces of which they are a reflection. This relates to the project of this book in that we should always be asking ourselves if our actions align with a liberal public health, or if we are establishing trends that take us in a different direction. This awareness can help us keep long-term considerations front and center each day, keeping our eyes on the ball of supporting a liberal public health. This is particularly important given how hard it can be to notice in real time when other incentives, such as partisanship or the pursuit of influence, are shifting our focus away from where it should always be—on promoting the health of populations, guided by science and reason.

Second, our focus on what matters most should permeate investment in shoring up the foundational forces that support health. It is not enough to simply be aware of the important if this awareness does not motivate an allocation of energy and resources toward engaging with these key factors. In the United States, we invest vast sums in health care, which is to say in doctors and medicines—which is to say into the urgent side of health.

Truly shaping a healthier world means creating the conditions where the urgencies of poor health do not emerge because we have attended to the important. The same goes for a challenge like climate change. In recent years there has been increased awareness of this issue, which is very much to the good. But if this awareness does not support greater investment in addressing the causes of climate change, it cannot truly make progress on this most important of issues. When it comes to addressing illiberalism in public health, this means not just keeping our eyes open, but acting, in the moment, on what we see. Many may disagree with the argument of this book, seeing no illiberalism in public health, but many may well share its concerns. Perhaps some of those who share these concerns have not acted on them, however, because they do not regard illiberalism as threatening the integrity of the field in the here and now. This is the wrong approach. Small threats in the moment can become big threats over time. This necessitates addressing these challenges as soon as we are aware of them, to deny them the chance to become existential crises.

Third, we should embrace a view of the challenges we face that considers both the urgent and the important, widening our perspective on the issues that matter most for health. During the pandemic, for example, we saw how inextricably linked the urgent and the important are, with the daily demands of navigating the COVID moment intersecting with broader issues. The crisis gave these links a clarity that they perhaps had not had before in the national conversation, motivating action to address the urgent by way of the important. This action included the federal stimulus package, demonstrations against racial injustice, and the choices of voters on Election Day. Looking to a post-COVID future, it is important that we maintain this comprehensive focus, with an eye toward averting slow-burning threats.

In considering the balance between the urgent and the important, my thoughts turn to a perhaps unexpected place: the works of Shakespeare. In his history plays Shakespeare is famous for commingling his depictions of great events—wars, social unrest, the crowning and overthrow of kings and queens—with scenes showing people's everyday lives and how their daily experiences were shaped by these broader forces. This balance is central to the vitality of the plays, to their capacity to fully reflect human life, depicting both the urgent and the important of our collective experience. Like a work of dramatic art, health is fundamentally a story. The way we tell it, what we choose to emphasize, shapes how healthy we can be in both the near term and the long term. When faced with looming threats, then, it is necessary to tell a story that captures health in its entirety, along with the forces that support it, so we can better act on the large-scale challenges we face while there's still time. This means working toward a liberal public health now, while the task is as manageable as it will ever be.

SOURCES

"Eisenhower's Urgent/Important Principle." MindTools. https://www.mindtools.com /pages/article/newHTE_91.htm. Accessed April 27, 2022.

Galea, S., and G. Annas. "An Argument for a Common-Sense Global Public Health Agenda." *Lancet* 2, no. 10 (2017): 445–46.

Keyes, K., and S. Galea. "What Matters Most: Quantifying an Epidemiology of Consequence." *Annals of Epidemiology* 25, no. 5 (2015): 305–11.

"Stanford Marshmallow Experiment." Wikipedia. https://en.wikipedia.org/wiki/Stanford _marshmallow_experiment. Updated March 13, 2022. Accessed April 27, 2022.

THE INELUCTABLE ROLE OF
THE FACELESS BUREAUCRAT

Much of the work of public health takes place within, and through, bureaucracies. From the institutions tasked with supporting health, to the academic world, to our work within national and global organizations, public health has long engaged with bureaucracy in support of its goals. Over time we have amassed significant influence within bureaucratic circles and have indeed used this influence to help shape a healthier world. At the same time, the nature of bureaucracy—with its insularity and lack of accountability—can facilitate illiberal approaches. It is worthwhile, then, to think about public health's engagement with bureaucracy, with the aim of aligning it with the liberal values that support a healthier world.

When I was in New York City a few years back, I commented to a colleague that much of the work of public health is about establishing bureaucratic norms. My comment reflected the way a core focus of our work is creating effective processes within institutions that support health—which is indeed the work of bureaucracy. My colleague responded by saying, "Wait till they call you a faceless bureaucrat." This remark—which I perhaps should have seen coming—captures the intrinsic disregard many people have for bureaucracy. The very word conjures blandness, redundancy, and red tape. This is reflected in representations of bureaucracy in film and literature—in the novels of V. S. Naipaul and Franz Kafka, and in movies like *Office Space* and the television show *The Office*.

So bureaucracy is easily lampooned. But exactly what are we lampooning? Is it the reality of what bureaucracy does or merely its *reputation*—the outward trappings of what is in fact a complex and essential sector?

In engaging with these questions, I realize I risk defending what many consider to be indefensible: bureaucracy. But if health is generated by the world around us, then bureaucracy—that is, the systems and procedures that organize our world—is *essential* to health. Hence it is well worth understanding these systems and how to improve them. This means first accepting that they do have a function, and a necessary one. I want effective bureaucracies to ensure that our system of roads and attendant regulations do not result in an unnecessary burden of accidents and injuries. I want effective bureaucracies that build healthy parks and green spaces. And I want bureaucracies that are resistant to illiberalism. Toward these goals, I will look at public health bureaucracy through the lens of its most recent test: COVID-19.

Within public health, the COVID moment brought the features of bureaucracy to light in different ways as we worked within bureaucracies to meet the challenge of the moment. During this time it would be fair, I think, to say that bureaucracy's record was mixed—that for all the good it did, it also made some stumbles. In particular, the following three challenges complicated our efforts to be maximally effective during the pandemic.

First, the bureaucratic structures in charge of communicating with the public at the national level struggled to do so effectively. While much criticism was rightly directed toward the Trump administration for the incoherence of its messaging around COVID, it is also true that the public health bureaucracy sometimes presented the public with mixed messages about what to do during this crisis. Bureaucratic messaging around the pandemic also could sometimes sound moralizing and pedantic, undercutting its effectiveness. This challenge of tone was perhaps informed by the tendency of bureaucracies to become bubbles in which policies and the terms in which policies are expressed come to reflect the words and priorities of the bureaucracy more than those of the population it serves. It was also affected by more explicitly illiberal influences, such as the wedding of scientific recommendations to political priorities within bureaucracies. This speaks to the broader challenge of when bureaucracies become, in a sense, their own constituencies, aiming to support their own internal continuity more than to achieve their outward-facing goals. We see this when public health gives priority to cultivating bureaucratic power and influence over its mission to support health. When we acknowledge this tendency, it becomes easier to understand how public health bureaucracies might choose to openly align themselves with political parties, judging it in their interest to do so.

Second, the messy rollout of vaccines revealed bureaucracy's limits in implementing solutions at scale in the midst of crisis. An organization like the Centers for Disease Control and Prevention can study vaccines, make recommendations about their use, even assist in their delivery, but there is only so much it can do to persuade people to get the shots. It is here, particularly, that the "faceless" character of bureaucracy can be a problem. The organizations making public health recommendations are staffed by people who were not selected by the public—this is true even in the White House, where just a handful of the decision makers inside were directly elected to their posts. This can produce mistrust—a feeling of "Just who *are* these people who are telling me to put something in my body?" This difficulty is perhaps less a failing of those working within the public health bureaucracy than a limitation of the structure of bureaucracy itself, one that has been on display during the pandemic. It also speaks to the importance of supporting a liberal public health when falling short of the liberal ideal can provoke mistrust of our efforts and make it more difficult for us to implement necessary measures.

Third, during COVID, bureaucracy to some extent lived up to its reputation of at times creating a chaos of rules and regulations. The pandemic was characterized by an ever-shifting fabric of laws and guidelines, shaped by the evolving nature of the virus and a changing social and political context. This context posed a challenge for all of us, of course, not just for bureaucracies. However, bureaucracy's structural predisposition toward complicated regulation and red tape made it seem, rightly or wrongly, less sure-footed than, say, the efforts of private industry, which did so much to quickly produce a COVID vaccine. (This is not to say that private companies don't have their share of bureaucracy. But companies are accountable to the demands of shareholders and the marketplace and so reflect a level of external accountability that many bureaucracies lack.)

I don't raise these points to argue against bureaucracy. On the contrary, a well-functioning bureaucracy, operating along liberal lines, is essential for supporting the public's health. It is also core to supporting our embrace of the public institutions that are the hallmark of a society founded on the principles of small-*l* liberalism. For these principles to flourish, the institutions that are their outward face must function in a way that inspires trust. To do so takes an effective internal bureaucracy.

What, then, does an effective bureaucracy look like? Effective bureaucracies must do what they're supposed to do, and do it well, fulfilling their basic operational functions (and, in doing so, raising the public's trust in the overall worth of bureaucracies and the institutions they support). It is perhaps significant in this regard that the military remains the institution Americans trust most, one in which effective functioning is nonnegotiable, a matter of life and death.

How can we ensure that bureaucracy does indeed maintain a high level of effective functioning? This question leads to a second feature of good bureaucracy: accountability. Organizations function best within an incentive structure that rewards effectiveness and discourages the lack of it. While bureaucracies may not be accountable to the voting public or the dynamics of the marketplace, there are a range of incentive structures that can be leveraged to support greater accountability. Then there are the demands of reality itself. Throughout COVID, for example, the demands of the moment have helped keep bureaucracy accountable by creating steep human costs for failure. It is when bureaucracy is most insulated from these costs that it is least accountable. In public health, then, the very stakes of our mission support a higher level of bureaucratic performance. In this way we can perhaps avoid the charge of being "faceless," instead remaining outward-facing, responsive to the needs of the communities we serve.

Finally, bureaucracies work best when they are not pedantic, embracing rules and regulations not for their own sake, but as tools to support health and improve lives. This means resisting the self-perpetuating cycles of red tape that can sometimes characterize bureaucracies, in favor of a flexible approach based on the needs of the moment. Core to this will be grounding our actions in the external data rather than in internal bureaucratic priorities. This can help undercut the charge of arbitrariness so often applied to bureaucratic initiatives.

Notably, all these suggestions have roots in liberal concepts of transparency, open debate, and democratic accountability. An effective public health bureaucracy, then, is one that is informed by a liberal sensibility, toward a vision of institutional functioning that is open, effective, and self-correcting in the face of error and new data.

As an immigrant twice over, I have had many encounters with bureaucracies, with real consequences for my future and that of my family. A defining feature of these encounters has always been a sense of whether the regulations and processes I engaged with were genuinely in place to support a better status quo for all, or whether they were arbitrary and redundant. With the former, it was always much easier to navigate the system. This supports a belief that bureaucracy should always be rooted in the work of making people's lives better, and that rules are meant to serve this improvement, rather than people's living to serve rules. We need bureaucratic systems to work well, and as easily as they can sometimes be lampooned, few of us would want to be without the services they provide.

SOURCES

Galea, S. Well: What We Need to Talk about When We Talk about Health. Oxford: Oxford University Press, 2019.

McCarthy, N. "The Institutions Americans Trust Most and Least in 2018" (infographic). *Forbes*, June 29, 2018. https://www.forbes.com/sites/niallmccarthy/2018/06/29/the-institutions-americans-trust-most-and-least-in-2018-infographic/. Accessed April 27, 2022.

SECTARIANISM AND THE PUBLIC'S HEALTH

Earlier in this book I suggested that public health's turn toward illiberalism is in many ways an understandable response to the rise of an empowered right wing, a political movement that has shown a willingness to dismantle the policies and institutions that support health. This has arguably caused us to view core issues in Manichean terms, with certain positions seen as on the side of good and others on the side of evil, with little gray area between. This is not always the wrong view to take. Some issues really are black and white, and when faced with a choice between being on the side of health and being against it, we have a responsibility to stand, always, with health. Yet it is also true that sectarianism has long been an ideal space for the rise of illiberalism, leading us to turn away from engagement and debate and toward a constant reaffirmation of our own certainties. It is worth asking, "In this context, if someone on the other 'side' had a good idea, would we even notice?" If some of their criticisms of us turned out to be valid, would we have eyes to see that? Likely, we would not. This makes it harder for us to correct our course when we are wrong and to reach out to the populations we serve, many of whom may not share our political views. Sectarianism in this way prevents the very engagement that helps mitigate the divides that keep our country sick, our politics unconstructive, and our approach to public health susceptible to illiberalism. It also encourages the politicizing of public health that has done so much to undermine our engagement with large swaths of the population. Changing this status quo requires a hard look at the problem of sectarianism, so that we might recognize and overcome the challenge it poses.

A 2021 Kaiser Family Foundation analysis found that Americans who at that time had not been vaccinated for COVID were three times likelier to lean Republican than to lean Democrat. The persistence of vaccine hesitancy had long kept vaccine uptake from being as widespread as it might have been, helping to prolong the pandemic. Its intersection with political partisanship suggests the role sectarianism played in this. Vaccine hesitancy was in many ways a product of mutual incomprehension. The hesitant, for a range of reasons, could not see why so many would find the vaccines safe enough to take. And the vaccinated, particularly those in the public health establishment, could not see why anyone would refuse an effective vaccine in the midst of a deadly pandemic. This divide mirrors other divides in the United States—most notably the sectarian red versus blue divide that has long characterized our politics.

This speaks to a key driver of sectarianism—our tendency to live in political "bubbles" where we rarely, if ever, encounter anyone with different views. Living in political bubbles can make it easier to mistake mere opinion for something that is incontestably, axiomatically true. It can also make it easier to demonize those who live outside our bubble, given that we rarely encounter them. In public health, for example, living in a political bubble is reinforced by a feedback loop: we stay in progressive spaces because we assume there is little of value in conservative spaces, which makes it less likely we will ever encounter anything to contradict our preconceived notions about their worth.

Notably, living in bubbles is not evenly distributed across the political spectrum. When we see antivaccine attitudes on the right, as well as an embrace of walls and anti-immigrant sentiment, it is easy to think it is the right that is doing the most to drive sectarianism. Yet analysis has found that the most intolerant county in the United States is in fact Suffolk County, Massachusetts—among the nation's most progressive regions. These data were a particularly rude awakening for me, since Suffolk County is where I work. It is difficult to admit we may be living in bubbles that limit our perspective on key issues, causing us to be narrow-minded without realizing it. Yet it is certainly true that we do tend to live in these bubbles, and in public health this can complicate our vision of the populations we serve. When we live in a bubble, we are liable to misunderstand the thoughts, feelings, and core motivations of the people whose health we would improve. This creates problems when we find ourselves having to ask these populations to change their behavior in some way in the name of health. Recent years have provided many examples of our assumptions about the population at large being off the mark. This was the case in both the 2016 and the 2020 presidential elections, when it turned out there were far more Trump supporters than many on the left thought. Perhaps even more relevant is that in 2020 Trump increased his share of votes among

Muslim, Black, Hispanic, and LGBTQ voters while losing votes among white men. The reasons for this are by no means clear. What is clear is that it confounds easy assumptions about race, class, self-interest, cultural affiliation, and political preference to such an extent that the only way to make sense of it might be to go outside our bubbles and engage deeply with the people we find there.

A core strength of liberalism, and one of the reasons it is essential for public health, is its capacity to foster such engagement. When we regard free and open debate as a core value, essential to the pursuit of truth, we are better able to do the hard work of talking to each other even when we vehemently disagree. If we dispense with liberalism, we will be left only with sectarian divides and little incentive to try to transcend them.

In bridging these divides, we need all the help we can get. Many of us would likely agree that such engagement is desirable, but actually pursuing it can be difficult, entailing pushback both from those we would engage with and from fellow inhabitants of our bubble. I experienced this in 2020 after writing a piece suggesting we need to think more about why President Trump's mishandling of COVID was not enough to bring about the landslide defeat in that year's election that many expected him to face. The implication of the piece was that our bubbles had blinded us to certain key realities about the country and the populations we serve. Seeing these realities more clearly will require the hard work of greater engagement, supported by a liberal public health.

Without this engagement, our efforts will be less effective than they could be, and we will continue to be at a loss to understand why. The challenge of vaccine hesitancy is an example of what can happen when stalemate settles in around the gap between public health's advice and how far populations are willing to follow it. We have a choice: we can accept the status quo as the best we can do in a hopelessly divided world, or we can embrace the hard work of doing better, even when this means engaging outside our ideological bubbles. We in public health must ask, Do we want to be open or closed, insular or a big tent that is inclusive of everybody? I would argue that the big tent is necessary if we are to fulfill our central purpose of supporting the health of populations. For us to be pro-health, we need a clear understanding of why some people seem to be so resolutely antihealth in their views. We should not engage with people we disagree with from a place of condescension, and we should not merely wait for them to stop speaking so we can communicate our predetermined message. Rather, we should engage at a human level, with the good faith assumption that there may even be something we can learn from those whose views strike us as self-evidently wrong. It is only by engaging in this spirit that we can hope to overcome sectarianism and advance a healthier world. Doing so is at the heart of a liberal vision of public health.

Circling back to vaccines, then, the more closely we look at the issue, the clearer it becomes that it is not so much about vaccines themselves as about the sectarian divides that underlie so much of our discourse about health. Because we have not yet done the work of healing these divides, their influence remains strong. Had we addressed them long before COVID, it is likely we would not have seen such vaccine hesitancy, a hesitancy inspired by a reflective distrust of anything that seems to originate outside a given population's bubble. This suggests that core to preventing the next pandemic is addressing the sectarian divides that have done so much to stop us from being as healthy as we could be. While this is a challenge, it is also an opportunity. The pandemic was a reminder that our health is connected, that the bubbles we find ourselves in are to a large extent illusory. They limit our vision, but they do little to keep out the broader context we all live in, which shapes our collective health. Stepping out of these bubbles puts us face-to-face with this context, which is where our attention should be, always, if we wish to build a healthier world. The key to doing so is through a liberalism that recognizes the importance of engagement both as self-corrective and as a means of generating new ideas and refining existing ones. If this liberalism is robust, we are well positioned to have the kinds of conversations about issues that might otherwise slip between the sectarian cracks. These cracks include the divides between people, groups, and—as I will discuss in the next chapter—nations.

SOURCES

Donnelly, G., and J. Kirchick. "The Increase in LGBTQ Support for Trump Has a Silver Lining." *Washington Post*, November 30, 2020. https://www.washingtonpost.com/opin ions/2020/11/30/trump-lgbtq-voters-support-silver-lining/. Accessed April 27, 2022.

Galea, S. "Learning from November 3: A Wake-Up Call for Public Health." *Milbank Quarterly*, November 4, 2020. https://www.milbank.org/quarterly/opinions/learning-from -november-3-a-wake-up-call-for-public-health/. Accessed April 27, 2022.

Habberman, M. "Trump Had His Greatest Loss of Support in 2020 with White Workers, Particularly White Men." *New York Times*, February 2, 2021. https://www.nytimes .com/2021/02/02/us/politics/white-men-trump.html. Accessed April 27, 2022.

Krizinger, A., A. Kearney, L. Hamel, and M. Brodie. "KFF COVID-19 Vaccine Monitor: The Increasing Importance of Partisanship in Predicting COVID-19 Vaccination Status." Kaiser Family Foundation. https://www.kff.org/coronavirus-covid-19/poll-finding

/importance-of-partisanship-predicting-vaccination-status/. Published November 16, 2021. Accessed April 27, 2022.

Miltimore, J. "The Most Intolerant County in America (and the Most Tolerant City)." Foundation for Economic Education. https://fee.org/articles/the-most-intolerant-county-in-america-and-the-most-tolerant-city/. Published March 15, 2019. Accessed April 27, 2022.

HEALTH IN AN ERA OF RESURGENT
GREAT POWER CONFLICT

In the summer of 2021, the journal *Nature Food* published a study that is in many ways a microcosm of a key force shaping the future of global health: the United States–China relationship. Notably, the study did not concern COVID-19. It was about soybeans. The study found that China's retaliatory tariffs on US agriculture could "cause unintended increases in nitrogen and phosphorus pollution and blue water extraction in the United States as farmers shift from soybeans to more pollution-causing crops." The study also looked at the potential global ripple effects of the trade dispute, suggesting that if China's soybean demands were diverted to Brazil, meeting them "may add additional pressures on phosphorus pollution and deforestation." Given how much our health depends on the condition of the natural world, these environmental consequences in themselves pose a threat to public health. More broadly, however, the force underlying them—simmering conflict between global superpowers—reflects an even deeper challenge to health, and to public health's engagement with liberalism, in both the near term and the long term.

In many ways these tensions are part of a larger story—that of globalization. Public health has long been engaged with this story, since globalization has increasingly helped shape the macrosocial determinants of health. As countries become more interconnected, their relations with each other have ever-greater influence on the determinants of health, both within and outside their borders. Rising tensions between the United States and China—fueled by a range of economic, cultural, and historical forces— have long been part of the conversation about globalization, but they have only recently factored into the conversation about health in a significant way. The emergence and spread of the pandemic were inseparable from the geopolitical concerns of the COVID-19 moment. From the start of the pandemic, the Chinese government was reluctant to share information about the virus, and the hostile posture of the superpowers helped maintain this status quo. This had consequences for our ability to address the

pandemic as it unfolded and to prevent future contagion. It also had implications for how we think about globalization, and health more broadly, in
a "shrinking" world. Great power conflict reminds us that health does not
occur in a vacuum, that it is shaped by global forces that are now coming
to the fore in the actions of great powers.

The resurgence of great power conflict may seem like a digression from
this book's core theme. In fact, few subjects could be more relevant to
the importance of supporting a liberal public health. Great power conflict is more than just a competition of economies and militaries. It is a
debate over ideas. The Cold War, for example, was in large part an argument over which system best supported freedom and quality of life for
citizens—liberal democracy or totalitarian communism. Tension between
the United States and China, while less clearly defined, echoes this core
question. China has embraced an authoritarian model along with the selected use of free markets, which has made it rich and powerful at the
expense of the freedom of the individual. The United States remains a liberal democracy that, for all its flaws, has done much to sustain freedom in
the modern world. Nevertheless, in the United States we have many deep
inequities that undermine our health. At the same time, China has inarguably improved the quality of life for millions of its citizens by creating the
economic conditions to lift them out of poverty. It also used its repressive
capacity to address COVID, embracing draconian lockdowns that would
not have been tolerated in more liberal systems. We know this because,
at the start of the pandemic, Western public health took cues from China,
basing containment strategies on what that country did and encountering
significant pushback from citizens unused to such heavy-handed measures.
Indeed, public health's willingness to base so much of what it did during
COVID on an autocratic regime was part of what motivated this book. It is
tempting to embrace some illiberalism during a crisis, as a means of more
efficiently delivering swift, decisive action, but such emergency measures
can compromise the integrity of our entire project as illiberalism takes
root in our field. A key risk of great power conflict, then, is that we find
ourselves becoming more like our geopolitical rival, letting our liberal inheritance slip away in the face of a dynamic, disorienting present. In public
health this means slipping even further from our liberal roots as we look
to more authoritarian models. While these models can seem to promise
greater efficiency, they do so at the expense of freedom. For these reasons,
we should consider public health in this new era of great power conflict,

with an eye toward navigating this historical moment without losing our liberal inheritance.

As the *Nature Food* study suggests, a resurgence of great power conflict has implications for health that extend far beyond the pandemic, intersecting with the full range of socioeconomic conditions that shape health. These include the economy, climate change, political shifts, and issues of war and peace—including the ever present threat of nuclear war. In addition, US–China tensions also reflect the national divisions we have seen between and within many other countries. From conflicts between Russia and its neighbors, to tensions between the United Kingdom and the European Union, to left-right divides here in the United States, conflict has come to define our era to an extent that would likely have surprised those envisioning this century thirty years ago, through the lens of post–Cold War optimism. These conflicts all inform the challenges of our time. However, great power conflict is something relatively new in the present moment, in these years after the Cold War, and is worth examining as a key challenge in itself, with many implications for health. I should note here that these thoughts are not meant to minimize the challenges posed by strained relations between other countries; these are indeed worth serious consideration. However, tensions between superpowers, with an explicit focus on the United States and China, are a distinct issue by orders of magnitude, and they are worth special attention to help us better understand what the dynamics of this issue mean for a liberal public health.

In the post–Cold War era, it can be easy to forget that great power conflict was once far more the norm than it is today. In Europe alone, the history of the past few centuries is in large part the history of great power conflict, with Great Britain, Russia, Austria, France, and Prussia/Germany all playing key roles and their relative power rising and falling as these conflicts unfolded. These conflicts have all helped define the socioeconomic context of their respective ages, which have in turn shaped health. In more recent years, conflicts have been smaller in scale, often taking place within states, between smaller countries, or with superpowers engaging in conflict with smaller states, as we saw in Iraq and Afghanistan. It must also be said that a key difference between the great power conflicts of the past and those of the current moment is the reality of nuclear weapons. These weapons, perhaps paradoxically, threaten the planet with annihilation while also helping minimize the chance of direct superpower conflict by raising the costs of such a conflict to a level no one is willing to pay. This can also prolong simmering conflict, as during the Cold War, by allowing tensions' to unfold without leading to the potentially decisive denouement of a full battlefield clash between superpowers, of the sort seen throughout the history of European wars.

Great power conflict in the twenty-first century is both a return to an older status quo and a new, historically unique situation with its own set of novel complications and risks, and with implications for health. What, then, are some of the key challenges that US–China tension poses for health in the near and long term?

Setting aside the obvious risk of open war, the most existential risk posed by resurgent superpower conflict is likely its cost to the environment— specifically, its intersection with climate change. Making meaningful progress on climate change will be difficult, if not impossible, if the United States and China cannot engage constructively on this issue. China is the world's largest emitter of greenhouse gasses, followed by the United States. Tension between the two countries complicates our efforts to solve this most urgent of problems, raising the possibility that even if this tension does not break out into war, it could still have dire consequences for the planet. At the same time, the environmental implications of everything from trade policy to the urbanization and industrial development of the two countries has ramifications for health. Leveraging these factors toward a healthier world will take willingness to work together toward the global common good, sharing knowledge and resources.

Second, great power competition poses challenges to the international institutions tasked with supporting global health. Global bodies like the United Nations, the World Health Organization, and the World Trade Organization help establish mutually beneficial norms of conduct for countries to abide by, and they help nations collaborate toward the common good. When these bodies become arenas for zero-sum competition, or when their functions are abused or corrupted by states seeking to dominate and bully, they cannot effectively support a better, healthier world. Shoring up the integrity of these institutions means working within them to ensure that the ambitions of great powers do not undermine the rules-based international order that is central to supporting health. It also means taking care that we ourselves do not embrace illiberalism within our own institutions, importing authoritarian models or simply turning a blind eye to the corruption that thrives in the absence of liberal norms.

Third, great power competition can make us want to retreat behind our borders, to emphasize geographic and cultural divides, and to turn away from the world's fundamental interconnectedness. COVID was a reminder that disease knows no borders. A health challenge in China can become a problem for the whole world in a matter of months. But it does not take a pandemic to show us how decades of globalization have created a world in which one country—particularly a superpower—can have an outsized influence on global health through its export of goods and culture. The United States, for example, has shaped the global diet, arguably for the worse, by contributing to the spread of fast food to seemingly the whole world. China, for its part, has been a key source of the fentanyl coming into the United States, fueling the opioid crisis. And the opening of Chinese markets to US companies has been inextricably linked to issues of free speech, data security, and corporate attitudes toward the Chinese government's stance on human rights—all of which have implications for the future of a liberal order that supports human flourishing and health. This interconnectedness, and its intersection with health, is inseparable from the context of great power competition. We cannot fully reckon with this if we retrench behind our borders instead of pursuing an optimistic, forward-looking vision of a global future.

Fourth, it is important to note that less well-resourced countries will likely suffer most from the consequences of great power conflict. This is perhaps best captured by the effects of climate change, which disproportionately harms low-resource countries in vulnerable parts of the world. It is also the case that, in past conflicts, the well-being of smaller, less influential states was often overlooked or undermined by the self-interested maneuvering of great powers. From the wars and economic exploitation Latin American countries faced as a consequence of actions of the Cold War superpowers, to colonial exploitation across the world in earlier eras, it is frequently the vulnerable who pay the highest price for great power conflict.

I raise these issues being mindful that there is no easy solution to them. The United States–China relationship is still very much in flux, its contours yet to be fully defined. However, in the midst of unknowns and facing an uncertain future, I believe that the liberal norms that have long guided us reflect our best means of navigating this uncertainty. This is particularly true when we find ourselves tempted to embrace the illiberalism modeled by our global competitors. While such an approach may indeed provide short-term efficiency, authoritarian competitors like China show us the abuses that emerge from such a system. An era of resurgent great power conflict, then, can provide a contrast worth remembering, readily clarifying the virtues of liberalism compared with its alternatives.

SOURCES

Agrawala, S. "How Low Income Countries Can Plan for Climate Change Impacts." World Resources Institute. https://www.wri.org/our-work/project/world-resources-report /how-low-income-countries-can-plan-climate-change-impacts. Accessed April 27, 2022.

Booker, B. "NBA Defends 'Freedom of Speech' for Employees as China Moves to Block Games." *NPR*, October 8, 2019. https://www.npr.org/2019/10/08/768225490/nba -defends-freedom-of-speech-for-employees-as-china-moves-to-block-games. Accessed April 27, 2022.

Felbab-Brown, V. "Fentanyl and Geopolitics: Controlling Opioid Supply from China." *Brookings*. https://www.brookings.edu/research/fentanyl-and-geopolitics-controlling -opioid-supply-from-china/. Published July 22, 2020. Accessed April 27, 2022.

Galea, S. *Macrosocial Determinants of Population Health*. New York: Springer, 2007.

———. "Trump's Careless North Korea Threats Obscure the Humans Who Would Suffer." *WBUR*, September 26, 2017. https://www.wbur.org/cognoscenti/2017/09/26/trumps -nkorea-threats-sandro-galea. Accessed April 27, 2022.

Galea, S., and J. Levy. "There Is No Public Health without Environmental Health." Boston University School of Public Health. https://www.bu.edu/sph/news/articles/2018 /there-is-no-public-health-without-environmental-health/. Published October 26, 2018. Accessed April 27, 2022.

"Hundred Years' War." History.com. https://www.history.com/topics/middle-ages /hundred-years-war. Published November 9, 2009. Updated August 21, 2018. Accessed April 27, 2022.

"International Relations (1814–1919)." Wikipedia. https://en.wikipedia.org/wiki/Interna tional_relations_(1814–1919). Updated April 25, 2022. Accessed April 27, 2022.

"Report: China Emissions Exceed All Developed Nations Combined." *BBC News*, May 7, 2021. https://www.bbc.com/news/world-asia-57018837. Accessed April 27, 2022.

Sacks, S. "Data Security and U.S.-China Tech Entanglement." *Lawfare*, April 2, 2020. https://www.lawfareblog.com/data-security-and-us-china-tech-entanglement. Accessed April 27, 2022.

Shultz, J., D. Sands, J. Kossin, and S. Galea. "Double Environmental Injustice—Climate Change, Hurricane Dorian, and the Bahamas." *New England Journal of Medicine* 382, no. 1 (2020): 1–3.

Swanson, A. "Nike and Coca-Cola Lobby against Xinjiang Forced Labor Bill." *New York Times*, November 29, 2020. https://www.nytimes.com/2020/11/29/business/economy /nike-coca-cola-xinjiang-forced-labor-bill.html. Updated January 20, 2021. Accessed April 27, 2022.

Yao, G., X. Zhang, E. A. Davidson, and F. Taheripour. "The Increasing Global Environmental Consequences of a Weakening US–China Crop Trade Relationship." *Nature Food* 2 (2021): 578–86.

"FOR OUR OWN GOOD"

When we were children, many of us were made to do things we didn't want to do. Our parents would tell us to eat our vegetables, or they'd send us to bed early or make us visit the doctor and get shots. They justified these actions with words parents have used since time immemorial: "It's for your own good." In some ways this phrase captures the essence of paternalism, which the *Cambridge Dictionary* defines as "thinking or behavior by people in authority that results in them making decisions for other people that, although they may be to those people's advantage, prevent them from taking responsibility for their own lives." Our parents' choices for us as children were our first exposure to this concept. In infringing on our autonomy they acted out of love, with the goal of keeping us healthy and safe. They did so because, as children, we were not yet able to make wise choices for ourselves. Because we could not always accept that our parents truly had our best interests at heart, we often resisted their efforts.

This dynamic unfolds in much the same way at the level of populations. We see tension between public health recommendations and a public wary of a "nanny state" bent on meddling in their lives. I have written about this before, participating in a debate with Leonard Glantz about the role of paternalism in public health. In that exchange, I argued that paternalism can be a positive force supporting the health of populations, provided it is informed by pragmatism and moderation.

I still hold this view. However, the context has shifted. In embracing a pragmatic paternalism, public health is tasked with using its power responsibly, toward the common good. In recent years, I would argue, it has fallen short of this task. During COVID, at times we saw public health use its power arbitrarily, without regard for the data. This was the case, for example, with lockdowns imposed even after vaccines and better treatments emerged, developments that should have radically altered our view of COVID-19 risk. I had some personal experience with this. In March 2021 my parents were under strict lockdown in a Toronto nursing home, despite having received the COVID vaccine along with all staff and residents at the facility. Their frustration echoed that of many in Canada and around the world who found themselves chafing at stringent public health measures that did not seem to be required by the data. From parents coping with ongoing school closures to small businesses suffering loss owing to lockdowns, many felt the burden of restriction during the pandemic. This burden could at times feel heavy-handed and capriciously imposed. This was certainly true for my parents, whose continued isolation made little sense once vaccines were available. It is perhaps ironic, then, that when we turned to politicians and public health authorities to justify these measures, we received answers that amounted to an echo of our parents all those years ago: "It's for your own good."

In public health, we support actions for the good of the populations we serve. Throughout the history of our field we have advocated for widespread hand washing, for redesigning cities to improve sanitation, for vaccination campaigns, for laws that restrict unhealthy behaviors like smoking and unsafe driving, and for changing cultural norms around a range of issues. These steps reflect "asks" of the public; we ask people to wash their hands, to put certain medicines into their bodies, and to consider new ways of thinking. And we tell them, "It's for your own good."

Public health measures do indeed, more often than not, support the common good, just as our parents' efforts to get us kids to do what we didn't want to do were in support of our own good. It's also worth noting that not all public health "asks" are onerous. In time, many are barely even noticed. How often do we think about the fact that no one can smoke in our office building, or that we must wear a seat belt, or that we were vaccinated as children? In most cases the answer is "rarely." Yet all these features of how we live now were at one time introduced to a world in which they were not the norm, advocated for by public health acting on behalf of the public good.

To be clear, there is nothing wrong with advocating for something for the good of a person or population. Nor is "for your own good" always an inadequate response to why a given measure is necessary. And as I've noted, I've argued in favor of paternalism when it's used in the right circumstances and truly supports the public good. Yet there are times when our belief that we are acting on behalf of the good leads us to embrace measures that are counterproductive to the work of promoting health. During the COVID period, I was struck not just that continued isolation for my parents and their peers made little sense in light of what we knew about the risk of COVID in a vaccinated population, but also that it was clearly harming their health. Isolation is difficult for anyone; it is particularly hard for older adults for whom time with loved ones is uniquely precious. Efforts meant to safeguard the health of older adults were, in practice, robbing them of the chance to make risk calculations for themselves. In keeping them sealed off even after they had been vaccinated, they were denied the opportunity to measure the diminished, but still present, risk of COVID against the certain harm of lost time with family and friends. This implied a lack of confidence in their capacity to make the right choices for their health, overriding the autonomy of competent people "for their own good." It also reflected public health's unwillingness to grapple with the trade-offs inherent in lockdown and isolation policies. Had we been better at weighing these trade-offs, we might have been better able to address the reality of what isolation cost older adults and the broader question of just how much we are collectively willing to give up in the name of safety—a question that is always implicit when we discuss paternalism in public health.

When our parents acted on our behalf, they did so because we weren't in a position to act for ourselves—we weren't yet old enough to understand the choices we faced. Likewise, when public health acts paternalistically, it should do so where a population is less able to advocate for itself. A good example is the effort to regulate the size of sugary drinks sold in restaurants. One way or another, someone will decide how big the drinks will be—and it won't be the consumer. The choice will be shaped either by corporate interests or by those acting on behalf of public health. In such a context, public health may indeed be acting paternalistically, but it will be in a way that affects the powerful, to support the individual consumer. It will be using power to constrain power, rather than using it to meddle unduly in the lives of those with less influence. This, to my thinking, is the correct use of paternalism, and this is not how it was deployed during COVID in places like the Toronto nursing homes.

In using power to override the autonomy of the vulnerable with no clear upside for health, public health was infantilizing adults who were perfectly capable of making their own choices. This infringed on their autonomy; it also infringed on their dignity. The idea of dignity rests on the understanding that each person has the right to make their way in the world while receiving basic respect. This aligns with the liberal principles of human rights and the importance of creating safeguards against power's ability to infringe on them. I should add that I have spent much of my career in public health arguing against those who say such safeguards mean we should neglect the common good in favor of unfettered individual liberty. Public health rests on the understanding that health is a public good, sustained by our collective investment in creating a healthier world. This means, at times, being willing to choose the creation of this world over certain individual freedoms. We trade a bit of the freedom "to" (to smoke indoors, to drive recklessly, etc.) in order to maximize freedom "from" (from disease and from preventable harm). There are a range of restrictions we have learned to live with. We do so with the understanding that they exist to keep us safe and healthy. It is also true that high-level choices are constantly made that shape our decisions about the products we buy, our capacity to live in pollution-free environments, our options for political leadership, and more. Given that these choices will continue to be made regardless of what we do, we should work to make sure they are made with an eye toward promoting health, for the good of the population.

This spirit animated much of the public's response to COVID. Despite the heated debate over various policies, we saw a broad willingness among much of the public to accept restrictions with the understanding that doing so helped keep us safe. This was particularly so in the early days of the pandemic, when we had little information about the disease, a vaccine was not yet available, and restrictions were being sold as a temporary measure. It was only when restrictions began to seem arbitrary, unmoored from the data, that "for our own good" started to ring hollow as justification. Compounding this was when the response to COVID infringed on the dignity of many who were already vulnerable—from older adults in nursing homes to children made to attend school remotely long after the data showed little risk of COVID in the classroom and significant risk in denying kids in-person education. These indignities run counter to a liberal public health that pursues reasonable, data-informed solutions with an eye toward balancing the relative harms of disease with the costs imposed by its mitigation. When we fall short of this liberal ideal, we risk projecting a tone that is condescending and reflects the worst kind of paternalism, alienating the populations we serve.

The solution is to recalibrate our words and actions in our pursuit of a healthier world. Rather than *saying* we are acting on behalf of the public's good, we should focus on *doing* what is necessary to promote health. We should speak with humility and act pragmatically in accordance with the data (which, if we are honest, we do not always do). And we should do this with the aim of getting better at weighing the trade-offs inherent in public health decision-making. This increases the chance that our "for your own good" asks of the public will align with measures that truly justify themselves in view of the challenges we face. As we saw during the pandemic, the public is willing to accept sacrifices if they are sure that doing so promotes health. Giving them this assurance means pursuing a liberal vision of public health that is rooted in respect for human dignity. We support dignity when we acknowledge the fundamental worth of our fellow human beings and our shared capacity for self-determination in the face of life's problems and uncertainties. When public health guidance—however well intended—infringes on a population's dignity, it should occasion serious self-reflection among those of us responsible for imposing it.

SOURCES

Galea, S. "Freedom 'to' vs. Freedom 'from.'" Boston University School of Public Health. https://www.bu.edu/sph/news/articles/2017/freedom-to-vs-freedom-from/. Published March 19, 2017. Accessed April 28, 2022.

———. "Paternalism and Public Health." Boston University School of Public Health. https://www.bu.edu/sph/news/articles/2016/paternalism-and-public-health/. Published March 13, 2016. Accessed April 28, 2022.

———. "Vaccines Can Give Older Adults Their Lives Back—We Should Let Them." *Toronto Star*, March 24, 2021. https://www.thestar.com/opinion/contributors/2021/03/24/vaccines-can-give-older-adults-their-lives-back-we-should-let-them.html. Accessed April 28, 2022.

Glantz, L. "A Commentary on Dean Galea's Note." Boston University School of Public Health. https://www.bu.edu/sph/news/articles/2016/a-commentary-on-dean-galeas-note/. Published March 13, 2016. Accessed April 28, 2022.

"Paternalism." *Cambridge Dictionary*. https://dictionary.cambridge.org/us/dictionary/english/paternalism. Accessed April 28, 2022.

Heresies

Shaping a liberal public health means facing the ways we have occasionally gone astray and grappling with truths that can be hard to hear—even when they go against the consensus.

WHY HEALTH?

Fundamentally, much of public health's struggle with illiberalism stems from a misunderstanding. It's a misunderstanding that speaks to the core of why we do what we do, a misunderstanding of a simple question: What is health for? There are two ways of answering this. The first assumes that health is nothing less than the complete absence of disease in society, and that this goal is to be pursued for its own sake, as an end in itself. This philosophy of health was the basis for much thinking during COVID-19, as many governments and health officials worked to eliminate all cases among the population, framing this as the central goal of their pandemic response. The second answer sees health as a means to an end. That end is living a rich, full, happy life. The aim of promoting health, then, is to enable as many people as possible to live such a life. Notably, a rich, full, happy life does not mean a life free of risk, nor does it mean a life that will last forever. It simply means we have taken reasonable precautions against disease and preventable harm and that these measures allow us to be healthy enough to pursue the activities we choose, in the company of family and friends. My bias has always been toward this second definition of health. It strikes me as truer to the fundamentals of public health, in which we aspire to create a context where all have the capacity to be healthy by accessing the resources that support a good life.

In recent years, however, it has also become clear that the alternative—the pursuit of an end to all forms of risk everywhere—can lead in an illiberal direction. To create a world free of all risk is to create a world that bears little resemblance to the one we have. It is to move far past reform toward a utopian ideal that, in practice, it takes a heavy hand to bring about. It also rejects engagement with the trade-offs that are core to realistic, data-informed decision-making. It is not surprising that many of public health's illiberal moments during the pandemic occurred in trying to eliminate all risk. Movement restrictions imposed against the will of much of the public, the policing of speech, tailoring our public health recommendations to fit the aims of our political allies and calling this science—these behaviors all become much more possible when our goal is to create a perfect world at all costs, one free of any risk.

Supporting a liberal public health, then, means engaging with the question "Why health?" It means being clear about our mission to shape a healthier world not for its own sake but for the better lives such a world allows us to lead. Why does it matter that we spend so much time working to generate health? Come to think of it, what *is* health anyway, at its core? What is it *for*? Perhaps in better understanding these questions we can better think how to factor in the risks we are, or are not, willing to take; to better address the steps necessary for getting to health; and to think better about the trade-offs inherent in any decision about the health of populations—now and in the post-COVID future. In doing so we can perhaps learn to sidestep the temptation toward illiberalism that can undermine our efforts.

Our behavior during COVID was therefore, in a sense, an answer to the question, What is health for? Before COVID, many of us might have said health is exclusively the avoidance of sickness and death. Yet during COVID we realized that, for most, enduring isolation was painful to bear, and even knowing that sickness and death were literally at our door was not enough to keep all of us from venturing outside. This suggests that health is, at core, a means rather than an end. It is a means to everything we were reluctant to give up during the pandemic: travel, time with friends, the pursuit of romance, furthering our education in schools and on campuses, peaceably assembling to advocate for social change, taking our kids to the playground, going out to eat. In short, health is a means to being able to do everything that makes for a rich, full life. Forgoing this richness might indeed help keep us alive, but few would argue that this would truly be *living* as it is properly understood.

I realize that suggesting health is a means rather than an end may seem to some like a radical rewrite of the nature of health. Conflating health with the absence of sickness is in some ways intuitive. Yet no less a body than the World Health Organization defines health as "a state of complete physical, mental and social well-being and not merely the absence of disease or infirmity." This definition reflects a long evolution in the way we think of health. Hippocrates, for example, regarded health as an equilibrium between the four humors—blood, yellow bile, black bile, and phlegm—that were thought to regulate physical and emotional well-being. This early definition bears little resemblance to the view of health as a means to the end of a full life, save for one important detail: both definitions prize equilibrium as the defining feature of health. To Hippocrates this meant a balance between the physical substances that make up a body, in which no single humor predominates. To the philosophy of health embraced by the WHO, equilibrium means a balance of the material resources necessary to enable the complete well-being of a rich, full life. Core to this vision is a definition of health that accepts the risk inherent in living such a life while rejecting the conditions that can make such risk undue. For example, there will likely always be some risk involved in riding in a car, and that is fine— that's life. But it is fine only if we have taken reasonable steps to mitigate risk, via seat belts, road safety campaigns, drunk-driving laws, and the like. The alternative path to safety would be never to ride in a car. This would keep us safe, but it would also mean never going anywhere. Embracing road safety creates an equilibrium that allows us to live neither ultrasafe in our bubbles nor needlessly facing risks we have the power to mitigate.

Public health does not always do a good job of factoring this impulse into what it says and does; we must improve at doing so if we are to engage with health on a level that does not conflict with our essential nature as humans. When we've asked populations to accept indefinite restrictions on their daily autonomy, implicit in our guidance has been the belief that the pursuit of health is an end in itself rather than a means to a fully realized life. We have often pursued a goal of near-total safety rather than of reasonable safety as a means of supporting living fully, with all the risks involved. Our unwillingness to engage with the trade-offs inherent in balancing safety with a reasonable amount of risk led us to take actions that could be described as illiberal.

COVID confronted us with the question, What are we willing to give up in order to achieve health? If health is the absence of disease and nothing else—if the pursuit of health means doing everything we can to drive risk of disease down to zero—then we are asking for willingness to give up much of what makes life worth living. As we have seen, few are willing to make such a trade-off for the feeling of total safety, even in the midst of a pandemic. However, if health is defined as an equilibrium, as balancing risk mitigation with the reasonable risk inherent in the pursuit of a full life, with health seen as a means to living such a life, the price for health becomes something more of us are willing to pay, and we need not embrace illiberalism to do so.

When we ask ourselves, What is health for? and answer that it is for enabling us to live rich, full lives, we are halfway to answering the even more fundamental question, Why health? Why does our engagement with the forces that shape health matter? Health matters because love matters, because connection matters, because working with valued colleagues matters, because tasting food matters, because going for a swim matters, because traveling abroad matters, because watching your daughter graduate from college matters, because living a rich, full life matters—which we cannot do unless we are healthy. To see health as an end in itself is too limiting to support the creation of a healthier world. It denies all else that goes into shaping a full life, even as it undercuts the work of public health by leading us to make demands of the public that they may struggle to fulfill and demands of our field that go against our liberal inheritance. The root of much discontent during COVID arose from the impression that health was being pursued at the expense of the conditions that allow us to truly live. A more moderate approach, which recognizes health as a means to this end, could well go further toward supporting health. If we truly believe health matters, our pursuit of it should reflect the understanding that we do not live to be healthy—we aspire to be healthy so we can live.

SOURCES

" 'And There's the Humor of It': Shakespeare and the Four Humors." NIH US National Library of Medicine. https://www.nlm.nih.gov/exhibition/shakespeare/fourhumors.html. Accessed April 28, 2022.

Basic Documents. 47th ed. Geneva: World Health Organization, 2009.

Conti, A. A. "Historical Evolution of the Concept of Health in Western Medicine." *Acta Biomedica* 89, no. 3 (2018): 352–54.

THE SPHERICAL COW PROBLEM

There's an old joke of which variations have long circulated. It goes like this: There was a farmer whose cows had stopped producing milk. The farmer tried everything but could not solve the problem. She tried altering the cows' diet, she tried putting them in a new pasture, she tried calling in the local vet—all with no success. Finally she took one of the cows to a world-renowned university in her state. The university was home to some of the brightest contemporary minds; surely they could fix her malfunctioning livestock? The professors were indeed willing to help, leaping at the chance to tackle a difficult problem. They agreed to examine the cow and apply their know-how to returning the herd to milk production. They spent weeks on the problem, making calculations, running various milk production models, and consulting researchers at other universities. When they had finished, the farmer returned to hear what they had come up with. Had they solved the problem? "Yes," said the lead researcher. "We have found a surefire way to increase milk production. First, let us assume we have spherical cows in a vacuum . . ."

This story pokes fun at the tendency of some who work in the idea space to embrace solutions that, while perhaps workable in theory, don't necessarily apply in the real world. The researchers were a collection of world-class minds, their methods cutting-edge, yet they managed to produce a solution that was, to anyone not ensconced in their bubble, not particularly helpful.

Having spent the past twenty years in academia, I have always tried to remember this story, hoping it can ground me in the real world, which universities are often far away from. In full disclosure, I've written my fair share of spherical cow papers, built on infeasible assumptions. But lately I have found myself coming back to the cow story more and more often, feeling that this is increasingly a problem we face in public health, where we are advocating for solutions based on theoretical assumptions that don't always meet the practical demands of reality.

The disconnect between our theories and the practical reality we must engage with offers a prime area for the emergence of illiberal approaches to public health. When our approaches are impractical, they are less likely to work. When they do not work, we are liable to become frustrated with the liberal framework that seems to be delivering these diminished returns—we may even become frustrated with the populations we serve for their "failure" to be helped by our ideas. This can cause us to move toward a path where we no longer try to suit our approaches to the realities of the world but instead try to make the world conform to our approaches—a clear route to illiberalism.

By way of example, let's return to a notion touched on in earlier chapters—"zero COVID." This idea, which made the academic rounds during the pandemic, suggested that we could get to a place where we reduce COVID-19 cases to zero. The general strategy was to create COVID-free "green zones" by eliminating the disease in certain regions. One by one these regions could then be merged, creating a country free of the disease. The fundamental idea, of course, was that we would expand ongoing social restrictions until we either eliminated COVID or achieved low endemicity. Now you may well ask, How could anyone find fault with such a goal? Weren't we all working toward a COVID-free world? Yes. But there is a substantial difference between using the goal of a COVID-free world to motivate success in addressing the disease and defining success against COVID as the complete eradication of the virus. The latter goal is easy to endorse in principle, but what are its implications? It would take lockdowns, mask mandates, and social conformity on a wide scale. To keep these steps from being ruinous would require massive government funding, vastly larger in scale than what had been devoted to mitigating the effects of the pandemic. It would take crackdowns on dissenting behavior and even, potentially, on dissenting views. It would have to include the cost of worsening substance misuse, drug overdoses, and poor mental health. And it would take focus away from addressing the health disparities exploited by COVID, as our pursuit of zero cases diverted attention from the more urgent, and doable, task of reducing cases among the socioeconomically marginalized communities the disease hit hardest.

I bring up the spherical cow problem not to suggest that public health is somehow out of touch or that we don't understand our own field. We do not suggest impractical solutions because we are detached from reality; on the contrary, we often turn to them from an abundance of data and a desire to apply our knowledge and good intentions to making the world healthier. But this very desire can at times lead us astray, turning us toward illiberalism. We sometimes misfire with our proposed solutions simply because that is where our good intentions lead us. The goal of zero COVID is attractive because it speaks to the kind of world we all wish to create: one that is free of disease. And as a long-term aspiration for our field, this is indeed the goal we should have. But as a specific benchmark for managing a crisis in a context of finite energy, resources, and political will, it has the potential to be counterproductive, a classic example of making the perfect the enemy of the good. Liberalism, with its emphasis on compromise and gradual reform, is partly defined by its steady but imperfect pursuit of the good. Illiberalism, on the other hand, often arises from the pursuit of the perfect by way of bad means.

In this context, zero COVID is arguably the quintessential spherical cow. From where many of us sat during the pandemic—in positions of relative privilege, working in the field of ideas—it made sense to embrace this slogan with all its implications. But this easy radicalism can elide the full complexity of the problem—the many shades of gray involved in containing an outbreak and allowing space for living, working, and the functioning of the economy. What is more, there is much in contemporary public health to discourage acknowledging this complexity. At a time when we had been thinking about COVID and not much else for more than a year, taking a nuanced view of how to deal with the pandemic risked appearing to side with the most reactionary forces in our society, even seeming to dismiss the disease. Yet nothing could be further from the truth. The challenges we faced in addressing COVID and mitigating its other consequences (on the economy, mental health, etc.) made it all the more important that we engage with the complexity of these issues. Anything less meant not thinking hard enough about how best to make it through a global pandemic with our world intact.

There is, of course, a case to be made that the point of calling for solutions like zero COVID is not so much to enact policy as to change the conversation around issues. Proposing radical solutions could be seen as a means of moving the Overton window—the window of acceptable discourse—in a more constructive direction; in this case, toward a more robust engagement with doing what needed to be done to protect us all from COVID.

But is there a cost to this? When there is a clear disconnect between proposed solutions and the lived experience they are meant to address, there is danger of alienating people who might otherwise join a coalition for action. For example, there likely are many people who supported taking some fairly drastic steps to ensure that no one unnecessarily contracted COVID but who were not willing to accept the notion that we needed to continue lockdowns when COVID was associated predominantly with milder cases and much less mortality. When abolishing risk was seen as a prerequisite for supporting a better status quo, many of these people opted out of the movement. By focusing solely on risk abolition instead of targeted risk reduction, we lost valuable time and support in our efforts to improve health. We also made it more necessary to embrace the heavy hand of illiberalism to force the conformity necessary to get to an idealized goal.

I realize these reservations may mark me as overly grounded in the world as it is, when the health challenges we face may seem to demand a more radical approach. But I am trying to reflect less on political exigencies than on the basic facts of human nature. When we feel we're being asked to take certain steps based on an incomplete view of reality, we are likely to resist these steps and distrust the people proposing them. When we propose solutions predicated on the existence of spherical cows and are not open to discussion, we don't just run the risk of looking silly. We risk being ineffective, illiberal. This is something we cannot afford.

Having said all this, I conclude with what is perhaps a twist: I'm not arguing that we should stop proposing solutions that call for spherical cows, I'm proposing that we stress-test them. I am proposing that we engage in dialogue about what solutions are possible, keeping an open mind about the plurality of perspectives that inform a liberal public health. This is consistent with our roots in the reasoned methodologies that emerged from the Enlightenment and that support the science that is the backbone of public health. We propose ideas, we test them, we adjust, we make progress. This is a pragmatic approach that has long served us well. There is much room inside such an approach for bold, far-reaching ideas, but only when such ideas are subject to change according to the practical realities of the moment. This means setting aside dogmatism for a constructive dialogue, often unfolding through peer review, to test our ideas by outside feedback. The public conversation about health is too important not to include as many passionately advocated solutions as possible. But its importance also demands we be willing to set these ideas against each other, to have a full and open debate about their merits, so that we may sharpen them and select the ones that are best. We should seek out counternarratives to our ideas, particularly when these ideas start to become orthodoxies. This means starting conversations with the assumption of good faith, even knowing that this faith will occasionally be misplaced. It means tolerating divergent viewpoints in public health, accepting that there is room for disagreement in our field, and recognizing that that disagreement, even with profoundly compelling ideas like zero COVID, must be grounded in reason and careful thought, aspiring to a better world within the bounds of what is feasible.

SOURCES

Horton, R. "Offline: The Case for No-COVID." *Lancet* 397, no. 10272 (2021): 359.

"The Overton Window." Mackinac Center for Public Policy. https://www.mackinac.org/OvertonWindow. Accessed April 28, 2022.

"Spherical Cow." Wikipedia. https://en.wikipedia.org/wiki/Spherical_cow. Updated April 4, 2022. Accessed April 28, 2022.

Stephenson, J. "CDC Warns of Surge in Drug Overdose Deaths during COVID-19." *JAMA Health Forum* 2, no. 1 (2021): 210001.

PUBLIC HEALTH AND THE
TEMPTATIONS OF POWER

My kids and I have loved the musical *Hamilton* since its music was first released a few songs at a time. At one point it seemed that my daughter had the entire music book memorized. One of the most memorable parts is the song "One Last Time," in which President George Washington announces his decision not to run for a third term, over the objections of Alexander Hamilton, his treasury secretary. The song's catchiness is a musical echo of just how notable it was when the real Washington decided to leave office. By that point in his career he was seen by almost everyone in the young United States as by far the preeminent figure of the age, and he could have kept serving, could even have made himself king. That he did not, that he willingly relinquished power after two terms in office, was both striking and celebrated. He has been compared to Cincinnatus, the Roman states-man who, after assuming the role of dictator to manage a military crisis, gave up power and returned to his farm once victory had been won.

Washington's choice to give up power ranks high among his achieve-ments, not just because of what it said about his character, but because of the legitimacy it conferred on American institutions. Had he stayed, the system would have become all about him, and while he may have contin-ued to do good in office, it would have come at the expense of the very institutions he spent his life helping to build. By leaving, and supporting a peaceful transition of power, he helped ensure that these institutions would remain strong and enjoy the collective buy-in of the people; a neces-sary condition for the functioning of a healthy republic. It was a profoundly liberal action, one that made the liberal ideals of the country's founding documents a reality in the United States, establishing norms that inform our political culture to this day.

Public health now finds itself at a similar crossroads with respect to power and its relation to liberalism. We amassed substantial power through our efforts to address the COVID-19 crisis. This was something of a change for us. In the past it was not uncommon to hear complaints that public health is sometimes neglected, that its recommendations to policymakers and the public can fall on deaf ears. The pandemic reversed this. Notwithstanding the polarization that kept a vocal faction of the population at odds with the advice of health authorities, we are in a moment when public health is more influential than it's ever been.

With the end of the COVID emergency comes the question of what public health will do with its newfound power. It's a sensitive question. We don't like to think of ourselves as wielders of power. In some ways, perhaps, public health is more comfortable seeing itself as the underdog; it's easier to imagine that our influence lies entirely in the data-informed efficacy of our solutions. But the fact is that public health has historically wielded power in key areas, and this power has grown during COVID. We are now in a position of deciding whether we should maintain this power at its current level once the crisis has passed or whether in doing so we risk the legitimacy of the broader liberal framework that supports health and the integrity of public health's efforts.

This is not to say public health didn't exercise power in these ways before the pandemic. We have long engaged with power in the interest of supporting health. Yet the pandemic has clearly expanded the role of public health, deepened its influence on policymakers, and amplified public health voices. By accepting this power, we were able to do much good. But this power also comes with challenges, risk, and new responsibilities.

It seems appropriate, then, to ask, What risks has this new power brought to public health? And how should we think of this power going forward, with the goal of minimizing the harms we do and maximizing our capacity to fulfill our mission?

To answer, let's examine the practical effects of how public health used power during COVID. At that time, public health worked with lawmakers to put in place protocols for navigating the pandemic. While these rules helped mitigate the spread of the virus, they also sparked backlash, as what seemed their arbitrary application led to challenges to their inherent paternalism. It is also true that we asked much of the population. While many diligently followed our advice, continuing to ask compliance when we knew it was no longer necessary risked shaping a public less willing to listen to us in the future.

By exercising power, public health, while doing good, also risks overreach, and the risk grows as the gap widens between what we ask of people and what is necessary for supporting health. Then there are the deeper risks posed whenever administrative overreach is paired with political power. We saw during the war on terror, for example, how the imperative of safety can lead to abuses such as mass surveillance. An entrenched administrative apparatus tasked with preventing disease through restriction, surveillance, and the shuttering of economic sectors could run a similar risk. The creation of such an apparatus was of much interest to Michel Foucault, who wrote about how the state's response to plague could serve as the basis for new forms of administrative control. Meanwhile, a more recent take on this comes from the Italian philosopher Giorgio Agamben, who expressed deep concern about the expansion of state power that can come with crisis—in particular the use of such crisis by elites to push through measures they have long wanted. That these concerns are to some extent justified is self-evident. We in public health, who could well be characterized as an "elite," have long worked toward the structural changes that shape a healthier world. As COVID exposed many of the conditions that make us sick, we tried to use the lessons of the moment as the basis for reforms we have indeed long agitated for. Put bluntly: we acted opportunistically in the name of a good cause, the cause of health. I don't think there's anything wrong with this; in fact, we would have neglected our responsibility had we done otherwise. However, we should be under no illusions about what we were doing, and how easily projects of fundamental reform, backed by state power and carried out with the best of intentions, can create the conditions for illiberalism and abuse.

We might well protest that we would never support abuses of power, that suggesting we could is so much conspiracy thinking. Yet history is full of examples of how the first step toward committing abuses is the unwillingness to suspect one's own motivations, as we assume that other groups are susceptible to the temptations of power but our own is not. This is arguably why we were able to amass so much influence during the pandemic without quite noticing how powerful we had become, even as we worked to retain this influence. The truth is that we are all vulnerable, and when we are occasionally accused of bureaucratic overreach and desiring to control others, the accusation springs not just from paranoia, but from a basic understanding of our common nature.

Finally, if we do not gracefully relinquish some measure of influence and control, we run the classic risk of power: corruption. Not corruption in the dramatic sense of, say, the scandals that topple politicians. I mean the kind that finds us compromising—in small ways and then, one day, maybe in big ones—on doing what must be done for health because it looks as if it might diminish our influence. It is human nature to become attached to power, even when it emerges from a crisis we all wish hadn't happened. We must guard against this tendency. As public health professionals, our motive must always be to support health. When we use power, it should always be in service of this goal, never as an end in itself. Keeping this in mind can help us avoid the temptation toward illiberalism.

I am stating this plainly because it is only by confronting the possibility that we may have become a bit too used to power that we can be fully effective in laying the groundwork for a healthier world. During the pandemic, the focus was on us, on public health. This focus was necessary; navigating the pandemic meant looking to public health as never before. The measures we recommended were emergency steps needed to meet the demands of the moment. But underlying the pandemic, always, were the structural drivers of poor health: the racism, injustice, inequality, and political neglect that create the conditions for poor health and that helped the virus take hold. Lockdowns, distancing, and mask wearing, so central to public health messaging and power during the pandemic, did nothing to fix these challenges—and they even, at times, worsened them by deepening inequality through economic disruption.

Shoring up the foundations of public health demands relinquishing bureaucratic power in favor of sustained collective engagement with the foundational issues that shape health. This work does not require a concentration of power in the hands of a single sector; it is diffuse, democratic. By placing the focus on health—not just on mitigating the pandemic, but on creating a world that is truly healthy—we can leverage our power toward the greatest possible good, by sharing it with everyone else who wishes to see a healthier world.

SOURCES

Caldwell, C. "Meet the Philosopher Who Is Trying to Explain the Pandemic." *New York Times*, August 21, 2020. https://www.nytimes.com/2020/08/21/opinion/sunday /giorgio-agamben-philosophy-coronavirus.html. Accessed April 28, 2022.

Lotha, G., Y. Chauhan, and A. Tikkanen. "Lucius Quinctius Cincinnatus." *Encyclopaedia Britannica* online. https://www.britannica.com/biography/Lucius-Quinctius-Cincinnatus. Published July 20, 1998. Updated June 19, 2019. Accessed April 28, 2022.

Miranda, L. M. (2015). "One Last Time." Recorded by C. Jackson, L. M. Miranda, and Cast. On *Hamilton* (original Broadway cast recording). Accessed via Broadcast Zero.

Hamilton: One Last Time [Video]. YouTube. https://www.youtube.com/watch?v=Pom CE3AQQEo. Published May 9, 2017. Accessed April 28, 2022.

Sarasin, P. "Understanding the Coronavirus Pandemic with Foucault?" *Genealogy + Critique*. https://blog.genealogy-critique.net/essays/254/understanding-corona-with-foucault. Published March 31, 2020. Accessed April 28, 2022.

"Washington—a Modern Cincinnatus." Frick Collection. https://www.frick.org/exhibitions /canova/cincinnatus. Accessed April 28, 2022.

NOT OUR PLACE

During COVID-19, public health made a number of statements that turned out not to be true (or at least turned out to reflect a truth more nuanced than the public health conversation at first acknowledged). These included the initial denial of masks' usefulness in slowing COVID transmission, an inflation of the risk of in-school viral spread, and a general favoring of indefinite lockdowns that obscured both the effectiveness of such measures (mixed, at best) and the socioeconomic harms they caused. In most of these cases public health was not held accountable for its missteps because there was no real mechanism for doing so. While political leaders must fear the ire of voters should they fail, public health officials are largely appointed rather than elected. For this reason, even though we often sounded like politicians during the pandemic, we lacked the corrective all politicians are subject to—the ballot box. In a sense, public health will always be to some extent insulated from the core mechanisms of institutional accountability. Not only are we unelected, but many of us are in a socioeconomic category that could be characterized, based on income and educational status, as elite. This can further distance us from the incentive structures that shape life outside our bubble and provide cover for our lapses into illiberalism.

It is, of course, not completely true to say there is no accountability for public health authorities. Our success or failure is measured by the most consequential metric there is—the lives and health of the populations we serve. Yet by the time the quality of our effort registers at this level, it can be too late to nimbly pivot our efforts—if they are indeed in need of correction—toward a higher standard of performance. It therefore is important that we remain self-critical, attuned to our strengths and weaknesses, so that we can make necessary course corrections well before our errors influence health for the worse. This means proceeding with humility, understanding that, while public health's "wheelhouse" is large—encompassing the full range of socioeconomic conditions that shape health—there are some places where our knowledge is less secure. This does not mean we should fear to tread where we are less experienced, only that we should be mindful that we are in a space where our knowledge is still incomplete. And in no circumstances should we act and speak as if we are experts when we are not. We should know our limits—know our place—or risk providing advice that is counterproductive at best, harmful at worse.

During COVID, we unfortunately did not always proceed with such care. The pandemic saw public health officials weighing in on all manner of subjects. Now, there is nothing wrong with free citizens' speaking their minds. Indeed, this is core to living and fully participating in a liberal society. However, the pronouncements of public health officials often were made in places like social media, where a data-informed comment on epidemiology could sit side by side with a tweet expressing, in an equally authoritative tone, the author's less well-informed thoughts about, say, foreign policy. This could make it difficult for the public to distinguish what reflected the author's true expertise and what was just opinionated spitballing. This matters for a liberal vision of public health, particularly because it speaks to a vulnerability of a liberal society. The openness fostered by liberalism means it can be hard to determine what is substantive and what is frivolous in the public debate.

What, then, is the public to make of this confusion? Ideally, people would take everything they hear with a grain of salt, obeying the old Russian saying "trust, but verify." But not all consumers of news and information are so discerning. During COVID, we often saw segments of the public either accept all information as the ironclad truth or regard it all as irredeemably false, depending on the partisan affiliation of the source. This led, in the first case, to much dubious advice being followed, not just by average citizens, but by elites in charge of important policy decisions. I leave it to readers to decide whether this is better or worse than the second case, in which segments of the public realized that in some cases public health voices were straying from their lane and decided, as a consequence, never to trust public health authorities again. The fruits of this were there for all to see in a robust antivaccine movement, anger over masking, and the demonizing of people with good intentions and deep expertise who just happened to sometimes give ill-considered advice.

In calling attention to this, I am not arguing against an expansive view of public health's mission. I have long been in favor of our opting for a wide-angle lens with regard to our work. I am saying we should be clear, and honest, about when we are speaking from expertise and when we are dealing with a subject we're still learning about. In doing so, we could learn much from those who have mastered the art of communicating a "work in progress" worldview in real time, gaining the public's trust precisely because they do not paper over their knowledge gaps with a tone of false authority. To find examples of this, we might do well to look in some less conventional places, paying attention to voices that resonated during the pandemic from outside the public health community.

Which brings us, perhaps inevitably, again to Joe Rogan. A subplot of the pandemic years was the controversy generated in the elite media over Rogan, the world's most popular podcaster, whose episodes regularly attract millions of listeners. Rogan would at times host guests who voiced opinions questioning mainstream narratives about COVID. There was much pearl clutching about how Rogan could have such a large following that clearly trusted him to provide better information than the legacy media. It's easy for the Rogan phenomenon to seem inexplicable when seen solely through what is written about him and through some of his more ill-advised statements. However, given his influence on the health conversation, it's worth listening to some of his episodes in full to better understand why he resonates with so many. In doing so, it becomes apparent that much of his appeal likely stems from his approach to subjects outside his areas of expertise. Rogan is an actor, comedian, and martial arts commentator who frequently hosts long-form conversations with doctors, scientists, philosophers, and politicians—in addition to his more disreputable, offbeat guests. This means he is frequently out of his depth. What separates him from many other high-profile interviewers is that he makes no effort to hide this. Rogan will often pause conversations to ask guests to explain concepts to him, sometimes quite basic ones. He issues corrections and responds to new information in real time, learning on the spot in front of a vast community of listeners. It could well be that he is trusted by millions not because he cloaks his ignorance in authoritative tones, but because he does precisely the opposite, deriving authority from a candid acknowledgment of his limits while working to broaden those limits, one conversation at a time. Might we perhaps learn from this?

I realize this chapter may be particularly challenging to the sensibilities of those of us in public health. We pride ourselves on our expertise, and to seem to suggest we should "know our place" is to appear disrespectful of all we have done to grow our knowledge and apply it in our work. Yet I am not saying we should know our place so much as that we should know when we are speaking outside the bounds of what we know best and, in those situations, should proceed with due humility. In a liberal marketplace of ideas, it can be difficult for the public to parse all they hear and easy for them to write off whole sectors at the slightest hint of unfounded authority. To support the viability of a liberal framework, we must become better at operating within it, tempering authority with humility and pride in what we know with awareness, and public acknowledgment, of what we do not know.

SOURCES

Powell, K., and V. Prasad. "The Noble Lies of COVID-19." *Slate*, July 28, 2021. https://slate .com/technology/2021/07/noble-lies-covid-fauci-cdc-masks.html. Accessed April 28, 2022.

"Trust, but Verify." Wikipedia. https://en.wikipedia.org/wiki/Trust,_but_verify. Updated February 23, 2022. Accessed April 28, 2022.

THE RADICAL IMPORTANCE OF
ACKNOWLEDGING PROGRESS

I tend to be asked to speak about problems, about challenges to health, and about the steps we can take to fix them. There is always much to talk about. As a world, we face many obstacles to health—from health inequities, to racial injustice, to obesity and gun violence, to climate change. These problems can seem overwhelming, and it's true that solving them is no simple matter. I have written and lectured often on these challenges, their scope, and the difficulty of addressing them. A core takeaway of this work is that it will take years of patient engagement to advance the structural changes necessary to shape a world free from the fundamental problems we face.

But it is also true that we have made tremendous progress in creating a healthier world. If given the option of being born at any time in human history, most of us would likely choose now. The world is less violent; people are living longer, healthier lives; more children are being educated; poverty has fallen, as has maternal mortality; and living standards have dramatically improved since the start of the Industrial Revolution. These improvements are fundamental to the way we now live. For much of human history, life was a brutal daily struggle for all but the most privileged. While many still live lives of desperate struggle, were someone from the medieval era to travel to the twenty-first century and see how the world has improved, she would likely feel she had arrived on a different planet.

As important as it is not to let our progress distract us from the problems we still face, it is also important that we not let our awareness of challenges minimize, in our minds, the tremendous, historically unprecedented improvements we have achieved. In previous chapters I have addressed how illiberalism can seem attractive when we feel we are in a moment of crisis. When it looks like our small-*l* liberal system has not delivered a better, healthier life, it is natural to look elsewhere for new ways of organizing ourselves. We are living at a time when it is particularly easy to feel we have made no progress. With a media and internet culture that emphasizes emotional, anecdotal stories over data-informed explanations of what is actually happening at the population level, it can be difficult to focus on the overall view of where we are. But the fact is, our liberal system has delivered progress—much—and the better we can see this progress, the likelier we are to remain invested in liberalism as the best way of achieving more.

Of course there is an argument to be made that it is not terribly important that we keep progress in view, that by downplaying our progress we simply avoid complacency, keeping ourselves ever invested in the work of shaping a healthier world. This is a powerful argument, but I think it is misguided. There is a short distance between downplaying progress and denying that progress is even possible. This is significant because, by insisting that progress is impossible, we are in a sense doing the naysayers' work for them by foreclosing the chance that any liberal effort toward a better future will meet with success, and making illiberalism seem perhaps a more reasonable alternative.

In arguing for acknowledging progress, I'm in no way saying that profound challenges and injustice do not remain. Studying these challenges is the key focus of my career. But I study these problems because I believe that by shedding light on them we can solve them. We can do so when we accept that solutions do exist, and that we have already made progress—in some cases tremendous progress—in their direction. Yet it has become seemingly inconsistent with a certain political agenda to say that we have made positive strides. Conversely, it has become untenable to many to acknowledge that the status quo is not perfect, that there are indeed problems to address. The conclusions urged by both sides are counterproductive: one side proposes to leave in place a status quo with many deep problems; the other side proposes to wholly dismantle systems— including liberal aspects of systems that may help to generate progress— because of a perception that the status quo is far worse than it actually is. In this situation, admitting progress becomes a radical act. It's strange to think this might be so, yet in an age when calls to dismantle systems have become commonplace, it has indeed become far rarer—and perhaps more daring—to say the world is actually, all things considered, rather good.

That we find ourselves in this position reflects both long-standing features of human nature and the unique circumstances of the moment we are in. As humans, we tend to overstate certain risks because, in the rare instances when such risks do lead to death or injury, the media has an incentive to amplify them to an extent that dramatically skews our perception of risk. On top of this, we now have the pervasive influence of social media, which can amplify an incident until it seems it is happening everywhere, regardless of whether this view is supported by data.

It's also worth noting that lack of progress creates a continued justification for the emergency measures that support public health's power. It's an uncomfortable fact that it's in our interest (when that interest is defined solely as maintaining our power and influence) that progress remain slow to nonexistent. While we in public health would likely balk at the suggestion that this plays a role in our unwillingness to acknowledge progress, it is nevertheless important to acknowledge that this could be a factor, if only subconsciously, in our discomfort with saying the world is better.

Acknowledging progress is made all the more difficult when our skewed perceptions fuse with our partisan affiliations. I was amused by an article in the *Guardian*, by Ed Cumming, headed "I hate to say it, but Britain's doing OK. Even Germany envies us . . ." The article's subheading is "For diehard Remoaners like me, all this endless good news about jabs and carbon emissions is pretty hard to take." The upshot of the piece is that, for liberals like me, who were (and remain) convinced that the United Kingdom is a lesser place in the wake of Brexit, the country's vaccination success, and progress in other areas, came as unwelcome news. The tone of the article is tongue-in-cheek, but it captures something true about what happens when our ideas about progress become linked to partisan affiliation: progress is particularly difficult to acknowledge when it seems to vindicate one's ideological foes.

At the heart of our inability to acknowledge and celebrate progress is our embrace of zero-sum thinking. We have come to believe that to acknowledge any progress is to deny all problems, or that to acknowledge problems is to deny all progress. We need to reject this thinking and reclaim nuance in how we see and engage with the world. We can simultaneously say it is a better time to be alive than ever before and also say we need to do even better—much better. One way to get to this perspective is to learn from those who are in a position to view our society from the outside. A good place to start would be with the millions of immigrants who have come to the United States, drawn by the freedom and opportunity upheld by our progress. I am one of these immigrants, coming to America as an adult after first moving from Malta to Canada as a teen. My immigrant experience has led me to see much of where America falls short, through my occasional encounters with bigotry and xenophobia. But far more fundamental to my experience as an immigrant is my deep love of the United States: its culture, its freedoms, and its liberalism. This love is why I am here. What's more, it is abundantly clear to me that my life as an immigrant to the United States is much better now than it would have been a century ago, even while it is clear that much could be better in our treatment of immigrants. I share this perspective being mindful that it echoes the thoughts of many others, who see this country through glasses neither rose-tinted nor focused on faults to the exclusion of all else. It seems important to say that we have made progress, that it matters that we have done so, and that we should celebrate this as we acknowledge there is still much to be done.

SOURCES

Cumming, E. "I Hate to Say It, but Britain's Doing OK. Even Germany Envies Us . . ." *Guardian*, February 28, 2021. https://www.theguardian.com/politics/2021/feb/28/i-hate-to-say-it-but-britains-doing-ok-even-germany-envies-us. Accessed April 28, 2022.

Galea, S. "Publications." https://www.sandrogalea.org/publications. Accessed April 28, 2022.

———. "Speaking." https://www.sandrogalea.org/speaking. Accessed April 28, 2022.

"Global Health Estimates: Life Expectancy and Healthy Life Expectancy." World Health Organization. https://www.who.int/data/gho/data/themes/mortality-and-global-health-estimates/ghe-life-expectancy-and-healthy-life-expectancy. Accessed April 28, 2022.

Roser, M. "Measurement Matters–the Decline of Maternal Mortality." Our World in Data. https://ourworldindata.org/measurement-matters-the-decline-of-maternal-mortality. Published October 25, 2017. Accessed April 28, 2022.

———. "The Short History of Global Living Conditions and Why It Matters That We Know It." Our World in Data. https://ourworldindata.org/a-history-of-global-living-conditions-in-5-charts. Accessed April 28, 2022.

Roser, M., and E. Ortiz-Ospina. "Global Education." Our World in Data. https://ourworldindata.org/global-education. Accessed April 28, 2022.

———. "Global Extreme Poverty." Our World in Data. https://ourworldindata.org/extreme-poverty. Accessed April 28, 2022.

"Study Settles the Score on Whether the Modern World is Less Violent." *ScienceDaily*, June 16, 2020. https://www.sciencedaily.com/releases/2020/06/200616113913.htm. Accessed April 28, 2022.

WHO'S LEFT?

In his inaugural address, President Joe Biden used the word unity eight times. Unity had been a consistent theme of his since the days of his presidential campaign, when he frequently said he intended to bring Americans together. Politicians often tout the virtues of unity, but Biden's message took on special resonance during the Trump years. The former president's willingness to lean into divisiveness as a political strategy—even, it sometimes seemed, as recreation—made Biden's call for unity a marked, and ultimately winning, contrast to Trump.

As compelling as is the idea of unity, however, the reality of political division is hard to escape. Division has been a constant in our politics since the country's earliest days. Accepting, then, that there will always be many sides to the American story, the question becomes, Which side is public health on? We aspire to improve health by shoring up the socioeconomic foundations of our country and the world. At the policy level this means a stronger social safety net, regulation of harmful influences like guns, and laws that help redress historical injustice. At present such policies tend to overlap with the goals of the political left. There are times, of course, when such goals are embraced by the right—as, for example, with the Trump administration's work on criminal justice reform. And there are legitimate conservative approaches to the issues public health tackles. But broadly speaking public health is aligned with the left, and there is no sense dancing around it. This is particularly true when the alternative is to have many in public health insist that they are nonpartisan while in practice they remain well to the left of the average American. Such a disconnect can look dishonest and undermine the public's trust in our efforts.

Defining public health's political alignment may seem tangential to the broader issue of illiberalism in public health. However, speaking honestly about our political biases can help explain much of the partisan thinking that has informed our work in recent years. When our biases lead us to take steps in outright support of a given political party, we risk letting science be co-opted by politics. When we do so, we leave behind the liberalism that informs scientific methodology and are well on our way to a postliberal engagement with the issues we face. Avoiding this means first acknowledging that we are indeed vulnerable to political bias and that this bias tends to favor the left.

What does it mean for public health to be "on the left"? The answer is not simple. Political alignment is tricky, taking on different meanings at different historical moments. Many of the positions that are currently mainstream on both the left and the right were considered fringe ten, or even five, years ago. Rather than parse policy positions, I would like to look at the left more broadly. Who is the left for? How inclusive, really, are our efforts to pursue a healthier world through a progressive political approach? I'm addressing the issue of inclusivity because it's at the heart of public health. Public health aims to improve the health of populations—of as many people as possible. Doing so means pursuing policies that are maximally inclusive, supporting the health of everyone and taking special care for the marginalized without neglecting the needs of the majority. At the same time, the effective pursuit of political goals requires the broadest possible coalition. So inclusivity also matters in that we should always be asking how well our approach serves the creation of such a coalition. When our political biases turn us toward illiberalism, we risk alienating the populations we seek to engage. Inclusivity, then, means maintaining a liberal public health, one that resists the politicizing of its work.

Inclusion has only grown more central to the left in recent years, as we have reached out to groups that have been marginalized in the United States, such as communities of color, immigrants, and the LGBTQ community. What's more, although the Trump years saw little in the way of policies benefiting these groups, they did see a shift in the progressive conversation as the left became more explicit and ambitious in its goal of supporting these groups through structural changes to the country. This is all to the good, yet we might ask, How inclusive has this approach been in practice? How has the public—and in particular the marginalized groups that are core to the left's political project—responded to the progressive call?

The results of the 2020 presidential election suggest some interesting answers. According to exit polling, Trump won a higher percentage of nonwhite voters than any Republican presidential candidate since Richard Nixon, and he doubled his 2016 support among the LGBTQ community. The reasons for these shifts are likely complex and merit exploring at length elsewhere. But it is worthwhile to reflect here on the fact that the shifts occurred among these groups in the context of a progressive movement arguably more focused on these communities than ever before. We may even consider that perhaps it was in part the tone of the progressive conversation around issues affecting marginalized communities that, ironically, may have driven more of those communities out of our coalition. At the very least, the results of the 2020 election should cause us to think deeply about our efforts toward inclusion and their practical political effects.

Of course, we may well take the election data another way, as an argument *against* inclusion, particularly inclusion of those who may not share all, or any, of our political views. It is easy to take marginalized groups' swinging to Trump as evidence that intolerance is insidious and widely internalized. It is also worth keeping in mind what is happening on the other end of the political spectrum. "Why should the left reach out," we might well ask, "when the right is in thrall to conspiracy theories, accepts bigotry, and regards the Capitol insurrection as a useful public service? Indeed, why continue to embrace a liberal public health when it has left us so vulnerable to these attacks? It's one thing to turn the other cheek to a slap, but what about when we see brass knuckles flashing our way? Isn't it better to put our guard up than to open our arms?"

These are compelling points. I would only respond that if we truly believe the progressive project is worthwhile—if we are serious about the policies that shape a healthier world—we have no choice but to advance an inclusive movement, rooted in a liberal vision. This does not mean compromising our principles—the changes that will get us to a healthier world remain radical, structural. Yet there is a difference between pursuing radical goals and doing so with the illiberal approach radicalism can entail.

By pursuing radical goals within a liberal framework, we may even achieve the elusive goal of unity. As much as we disagree, everyone desires health; if there was ever an aspiration that could bring people together, it's surely the wish to be healthy. In public health, we well understand the harm divisions can create, how they inform the health gaps that keep our society sick. Uniting people around the common goal of health could help end the sickness we've seen so much of. For this reason, as we engage with the left we in public health have a special responsibility to occasionally look beyond it, toward the aim of better health for everyone. This will require us to be generous in our embrace of others and to see beyond divides. We cannot do this when we are pursuing a healthier world using illiberal means. Core to liberalism is openness, the creation of a public square where we can all be heard. Turning our back on this ideal will cause us to fall short of true inclusion and to embrace a vision of public health that is less sustainable than it otherwise would be.

A quotation from Khaled Hosseini says, "One is well served by a degree of both humility and charity when judging the inner working of another person's heart." This is, I think, a sound basis on which to engage with others, especially in an age when it has never been easier to object to what our neighbors think and say. Liberalism calls on us to turn toward our neighbors and away from our biases, to prioritize the common good over a particular point of view, and to have the humility to place skepticism and science above ideological certainty.

So can we in public health lead the way? Can we show the world that it is better, healthier, if we explicitly let go of always taking sides, because we know these divisions harm health? Until we can answer yes to these questions, we cannot be effective enough in navigating this moment. Getting to yes means embracing a liberal vision of public health that can indeed accommodate different points of view, rather than the zero-sum engagement of a purely partisan focus.

SOURCES

Allen, M. "Biden Pushes Unity Message in New TV Wave." *Axios*, September 25, 2020. https://www.axios.com/biden-unity-message-campaign-ad-02ef11e3-9732-4753-b1f0 -37f72b876188.html. Accessed April 28, 2022.

Gallo, C. "This Is What Made President Joe Biden's Inauguration Speech So Powerful." *Forbes*, January 20, 2021. https://www.forbes.com/sites/carminegallo/2021/01/20/joe -biden-inauguration-speech-an-american-story-of-hope/. Accessed April 28, 2022.

Hosseini, K. Quotation by Khaled Hosseini. Goodreads. https://www.goodreads.com /quotes/7095029-one-is-well-served-by-a-degree-of-both-humility. Accessed April 28, 2022.

Impelli, M. "Trump Wins Highest Percent of Nonwhite Voters of Any Republican in 60 Years, Doubles LGBTQ Support from 2016: Exit Poll." *Newsweek*, November 5, 2020. https://www.newsweek.com/trump-wins-highest-percent-nonwhite-voters-any -republican-60-years-doubles-lgbtq-support-2016-1545294. Accessed April 28, 2022.

Lopez, G. "The First Step Act, Explained." *Vox*. https://www.vox.com/future-perfect /2018/12/18/18140973/state-of-the-union-trump-first-step-act-criminal-justice-reform. Updated February 5, 2019. Accessed April 28, 2022.

McWhorter, J. "The Black People Who Voted for Trump Know He's Racist." *Atlantic*, September 16, 2020. https://www.theatlantic.com/ideas/archive/2020/11/racism-isnt -everyones-priority/617108/. Accessed April 28, 2022.

Montanaro, D. "Biden Eschews Anger, Hoping 'Unity' Can Lift Him to the Presidency." *NPR*, May 19, 2019. https://www.npr.org/2019/05/19/724708438/biden-eschews -anger-hoping-unity-can-lift-him-to-the-presidency. Accessed April 28, 2022.

Spocchia, G. "45% of Republicans Approve of the Capitol Riots, Poll Claims." *Indepen-dent*, January 7, 2021. https://www.independent.co.uk/news/world/americas/us -election-2020/republicans-congress-capitol-support-trump-b1783807.html. Accessed April 28, 2022.

TOO FAR, OR NOT FAR ENOUGH?

The business of creating a healthier world is fundamentally the business of pushing for change. This means pushing against a status quo that often does not serve us well. It can require us to oppose systems, and even people, that are invested in entrenching the drivers of poor health. This is all to the good. However, while we are quite familiar with the reasons this pushing is necessary—an awareness informed by our understanding of the drivers of poor health—less discussed are some of the ways this pursuit of change can at times undermine itself, leading in counterproductive directions. This is well illustrated through a story told by the conservative political theorist Kenneth Minogue, one he used to critique the development of liberalism:

> The story of liberalism, as liberals tell it, is rather like the legend of St. George and the dragon. After many centuries of hopelessness and superstition, St. George, in the guise of Rationality, appeared in the world somewhere about the sixteenth century. The first dragons upon whom he turned his lance were those of despotic kingship and religious intolerance. These battles won, he rested for a time, until such questions as slavery, or prison conditions, or the state of the poor, began to command his attention. During the nineteenth century, his lance was never still, prodding this way and that against the inert scaliness of privilege, vested interest, or patrician insolence. But, unlike St. George, he did not know when to retire. The more he succeeded, the more he became bewitched with the thought of a world free of dragons, and the less capable he became of ever returning to private life. He *needed* his dragons. He could only live by fighting for causes—the people, the poor, the exploited, the colonially oppressed, the underprivileged and the underdeveloped. As an ageing warrior, he grew breathless in his pursuit of smaller and smaller dragons—for the big dragons were now harder to come by.

I acknowledge that this story, excerpted from Minogue's book *The Liberal Mind*, may strike some readers as unfair. Where Minogue sees "smaller dragons," a different perspective might see normal-sized dragons that we are just now giving the correct measure of attention.

Yet it is hard to deny that Minogue's story raises some necessary, though perhaps uncomfortable, questions: Do we too in some degree *need* our dragons, even if certain challenges have diminished or changed over time? Can we know progress when we see it, and, if not, what forces may be clouding our vision? If, in our pursuit of smaller dragons, we come to believe that a dragonless world is simply not possible within a liberal context, will we turn to an illiberal alternative? Avoiding this illiberalism means recognizing when our pursuit of a better world tempts us to go too far, to lose perspective in our zeal to make progress. When we mistake small dragons for big ones, we are more likely to embrace measures that are out of proportion to the threats we face, and that may backfire by corrupting our mission, lessening our ability to act as a force for good.

How, then, can we stop ourselves from going too far, from embracing illiberalism in our hunt for dragons? The best way to start is by revisiting core questions: Just what are we trying to achieve in public health? How would we like to align the world so that it best supports health? I think that within the public health community there is broad consensus on what such a world would look like. At a fundamental level, it would be characterized by social and economic justice. By economic justice, I mean a world where economic systems are geared toward fairness rather than the inequality that currently benefits the well-off few at the expense of the less well-off many. By social justice, I mean a world where no one is unfairly held back by characteristics of identity—whether race, sexual orientation, or gender.

Having established these goals, we might then ask, What are the key impediments to the fundamental socioeconomic realignments it will take to achieve them? For those who have long engaged with progressive work, the answer will likely include something along the lines of corporate interests, reactionary political movements, public apathy, and deep-rooted societal pathologies like racism, homophobia, and misogyny. Calibrating our efforts toward a healthier future must, as a practical matter, consider resistance from these areas, these familiar dragons. Over the past few years we have seen a more explicit, even confrontational engagement with these forces, which has arguably elevated the public's awareness of the foundational forces that shape our lives and health, even as it has occasionally tempted us to go too far, to act illiberally.

Insofar as this invigorated engagement has advanced the goal of progressive change, I would say it has been to the good, doing much to shape a necessary realignment. But this engagement, for all the good it has done, also raises a potential impediment to positive change. The problems that stand in the way of a healthier world are not to be solved overnight; thus our push for change has given rise to organizations, fundraising networks, and, indeed, a professional activism that aims to sustain momentum over the long term. This is now a sector in itself, one that would not exist without the presence of challenges in our world. It is also true that pushing for positive change can bring many rewards, such as the appearance of virtue and the social currency that comes with being on what is widely regarded as the right side of an issue. All this has created an incentive structure where those who push for change, in fact, have much to gain by nothing's changing. This can lead to our becoming much like Saint George and the dragon. As we make key gains in the work of building a healthier world, there is a temptation to apply to less significant challenges the same level of intensity and moral force we apply to more clearly existential threats, to justify an activism whose tone is that of a knight constantly charging into battle. There is even the risk that we will continue to value our power and influence above achieving the successes we claim to want in our pursuit of a healthier world. This is not to say, of course, that those pushing for change would ever consciously wish for injustice to continue. But it would be naive to deny there are incentives in place that might keep Saint George in the workforce, using the same skills as ever, regardless of how the issues that shape health evolve. Within a liberal framework, we can recognize this and work to correct our course. Within an illiberal paradigm, however, we need not trouble ourselves with such a contradiction; we may even embrace it as a means of perpetuating our own power and influence.

How then can we properly calibrate our work to ensure that we always meet the moment but do not overshoot crises and risk prolonging them, tipping ourselves into illiberalism in the process? I think we can do so through three key steps.

First, if we wish to change systems, we need to become better at understanding the perspectives of those who do not share our approach. At a practical level, this can help achieve the mutual understanding that can support new areas of collaboration. Perhaps more significantly, engaging in good faith with those who may not share our goals can make us examine our own motives, giving us the perspective that can help us see when we may need to recalibrate our approach to challenges. Such engagement is well facilitated by a liberal framework.

Second, we can remember that, when it seems our work calls for up-ending systems, we should not pursue this course lightly, nor should we do so without first considering different approaches to the problems at hand. When confronted with challenges, the temptation is to be quick to embrace upending systems as the go-to solution for all problems, discarding the liberalism that sustains these systems without pausing to consider other options. Now, changing systems often is indeed the right way to address problems. Indeed, I left practicing medicine to work in public health because I saw pushing for systemic change as the key to generating health on a large scale. But there is also truth to the old saying that to a hammer everything looks like a nail, so activism committed to bold change should be willing to check its motivations, to be sure its proposed solutions fit what the moment calls for. To answer every challenge with a call for complete upheaval of all that came before is to be neither serious nor effective as a movement.

Third, we can take care to calibrate our words according to the needs of the moment. We may not want to use the language of overthrow when pragmatic reform is called for, just as we may not want to talk about incremental reform when our speech might support something bolder. If we continually cry "revolution" when we really need basic, commonsense reforms, we are liable to drive otherwise sympathetic partners out of our coalition. We also risk being taken less seriously when systemic change really is necessary, with our calls for bold action falling on ears that have long since ceased to listen. If, on the other hand, we always shy away from calling for boldness, we are clearly falling short, in a different way, of our mission to advance the structural change that supports health. Rather than going too far, or not far enough, what we need is balance and a willingness to speak with care and precision about the issues at hand. It is also worth noting that boldness and liberalism are not mutually exclusive. Our system is flexible enough to accommodate revolution and reaction in equal measure, as long as both observe the rules of the game. It's when we find ourselves reaching to sweep these rules aside that we risk going too far.

SOURCES

Galea, S. "A Case for Good Faith Argument." *Healthiest Goldfish* (blog), May 29, 2021. https://sandrogalea.substack.com/p/a-case-for-good-faith-argument. Accessed April 28, 2022.

————. "The Radical Importance of Acknowledging Progress." *Healthiest Goldfish* (blog),
   April 30, 2021. https://sandrogalea.substack.com/p/the-radical-importance-of
   -acknowledging. Accessed April 28, 2022.
Minogue, K. R. "Quotation by Kenneth Minogue." Goodreads. https://www.goodreads
   .com/quotes/838011-the-story-of-liberalism-as-liberals-tell-it-is-rather. Accessed
   April 28, 2022.
————. *The Liberal Mind*. Indianapolis, IN: Liberty Fund; 2001.

A CASE AGAINST MORALISM
IN PUBLIC HEALTH

Throughout this book so far, I have alluded to the importance of tone in public health messaging. How we engage with the public plays a key role in how the public engages with us. When we appear to moralize, trying to finger-wag our way to a healthier world, the public may tune us out. This in turn increases the chance that we will turn toward illiberalism, seeking to impose public health measures where before we had tried to persuade people to accept them. For this reason, it's worth taking a moment to focus on our tone and, in particular, on our tendency to come across as moralizing—a tone that can verge on the outright stigmatizing of segments of the populations we serve.

Public health has long had an uneasy relationship with scapegoating and stigma. We generally oppose them, understanding that they inform the marginalizing that creates health gaps and limits the scope of prevention efforts. Yet the truth is that we selectively embrace stigma when we think doing so will support health. The classic example is smoking. Smoking has declined over the past fifty years because of greater regulation of the tobacco industry, but also because it has become socially unacceptable. That it is now so regarded is due, in part, to public health's willingness to make explicit the risks that smokers impose not just on themselves, but on communities. Put simply, we have embraced stigmatizing a certain behavior in the name of the common good. Smoking kills, and we have spent the past fifty years making sure as many people as possible know it. This knowledge is now so common that there is indeed a case to be made that those who smoke these days knowingly put themselves and others at risk. We can now plausibly say the choice to smoke or not smoke is, in a sense, a choice between right and wrong.

The same was to some extent true of COVID-19. We *did* know that wearing masks and limiting our physical interaction would reduce the spread of the disease. Taking these steps was—there's no getting around it—a matter of personal responsibility, a moral consideration, and it was right for us to acknowledge this.

But there is also real peril in a public health approach steeped in moralism. Such an approach can overlook the conditions that constrain people's lives and choices. Just as we should not ignore personal responsibility, we should not ignore the way factors like employment, income, education level, and neighborhood affect people's ability to choose health. Part of our liberal inheritance is maintaining an inclusive public debate in which all perspectives have a seat at the table. If we ignore the populations whose lives are shaped by conditions different from those that shape our own, we are acting contrary to the spirit of liberalism. COVID provided many examples of how such conditions create gaps in the lived experience of populations. We know, for example, that there is a clear link between income quartile and ability to physically distance by working remotely. Data from the Bureau of Labor Statistics has shown that 62 percent of earners in the top twenty-fifth quartile were able to work remotely, compared with just 9 percent of those in the bottom twenty-fifth. Messaging that shames people for not staying home, then, may drive away the very populations we aim to protect and push us toward an illiberal approach to health.

The implication here is that in stigmatizing those who do not adhere to physical distancing protocols, we risk targeting those with the least personal control over whether they do so. We also know that stigmatizing behavior can be harmful in itself. In 2009 I worked with Jennifer Stuber and Bruce Link on a study of smoking and stigma. We found that smoking-related stigma, however good the intentions behind it, can have a negative influence on well-being, particularly when it encourages secrecy and social withdrawal owing to feeling devalued by society for one's choices.

Then there is the important question of whether stigma actually does encourage healthier behavior. I'm not so sure it does. The data on the efficacy of behavioral modification interventions are dubious. Indeed, there is evidence that overly negative public health advertising can sometimes be less effective. At the very least, getting public health messaging right is a complex task, ill served by "one size fits all" approaches. People are complicated, and using shame as a cudgel will not always have the desired effect.

This approach can backfire. Let's take as a case study one of the most important efforts that public health is tackling right now: addressing deeply rooted systems of racial inequity and injustice. That structural racism is a real and present threat to the health of the public is inarguable. That we should be tackling this challenge head-on is equally so. But one approach that has been adopted in many organizations, to the exclusion of real engagement with harder, deeper challenges, has been workplace diversity programs. These have proliferated in the past decade. Such programs have been widely adopted out of the best possible motives—to address bias, promote understanding across barriers of perceived difference, and create more inclusive work environments where everyone can thrive. Implicit in hosting these programs is the acknowledgment that bias is deeply undesirable and that anyone supporting such bias is on the wrong side not just of company policy, but of morality. This raises the stakes considerably, as it should. Workplace bias, incidents of bigotry, and discriminatory systems have no place in a functional organization or, indeed, in a healthy society. Yet data suggest that diversity programs are not always effective at changing behavior and can at times actually reinforce bias. This result can be a consequence of participants' chafing at what they can see as a coercive element to the training—an element that reflects the illiberalism that can creep in when we impose measures "for your own good."

To reiterate: such deeper engagement with racism, and its structural effects, is very much to the good—in fact it is critical to our mission. The work of public health is in large part the work of understanding how our country's racial history has created systemic disadvantage for communities of color. At the same time, an approach to addressing the systems underlying racial injustice that leads with condemnation, that overlooks the individuals at the heart of systems, and that minimizes the critical role of mercy and forgiveness risks undermining the broader goals of justice-oriented change movements. Moralism may indeed be useful in encouraging healthier behaviors, but only when coupled with true compassion and the understanding that we in public health are not exempt from the standards to which we hold others. Moralism, to be effective, may need mercy in parallel. With this in mind we should tread lightly, particularly when we are most tempted to take a harder line.

This is, I suggest, particularly important in our current moment, when virtue is often confused with "virtue signaling," a confusion encouraged by the incentives of social media. Online it is easy to criticize, to condemn, and to feel righteous for sounding "good" or virtuous. The question we must ask is, What is this approach actually accomplishing? Is it advancing the cause of a healthier world? Or are we merely spinning our wheels? Or, worse, are we actively setting our cause back by sowing the seeds of backlash rather than doing the harder, but arguably more effective, work of reaching out to others in full awareness of the complexity of their lives and motivations, then engaging from a place of humility and good faith? It is also worth asking if, given the power of media feedback loops, we even fully notice the moralizing tone we sometimes strike. Are we truly hearing ourselves? If so, can we honestly say we always like the way we sound?

It's necessary to pose these questions, and to answer them honestly, because it's necessary that public health be seen as credible, particularly in a time of crisis. If it isn't, if people tune us out or reflexively do the opposite of what we recommend simply because they don't like us, then it doesn't matter what knowledge we generate, what clever solutions we propose, or how firmly on the right side of history we feel we are (even as we may compromise our position by turning to illiberalism)—our efforts will fail. We will be seen not as figures to be trusted, but as priggish moralizers or tiresome pedants.

There is a stock character in commedia dell'arte known as *Il Dottore*. He is a classic pedant, a parody of educated elites: well read, decadent, verbose, and stuffed with useless knowledge—useless because no one takes him seriously. We cannot afford to be him. When public health is dismissed it is ineffectual, and when it is ineffectual, people sicken and die. Moralizing may make us feel right—it may even allow us to feel effective—but in the end it does no favors for health.

SOURCES

Chang, E. H., K. L. Milkman, D. M. Gromet, et al. "The Mixed Effects of Online Diversity Training." *Proceedings of the National Academy of Sciences of the United States of America* 116, no. 16 (2019): 7778–83.

Chang, E. H., K. L. Milkman, L. J. Zarrow, et al. "Does Diversity Training Work the Way It's Supposed To?" *Harvard Business Review*, July 9, 2019. https://hbr.org/2019/07/does-diversity-training-work-the-way-its-supposed-to. Accessed April 28, 2022.

"Cigarette Smoking among U.S. Adults Hits All-Time Low." Centers for Disease Control and Prevention. https://www.cdc.gov/media/releases/2019/p1114-smoking-low.html. Accessed April 28, 2022.

Dobbin, F., and A. Kalev. "Why Diversity Programs Fail." *Harvard Business Review*, July-August 2016. https://hbr.org/2016/07/why-diversity-programs-fail. Accessed April 28, 2022.

"Il Dottore." Wikipedia. https://en.wikipedia.org/wiki/Il_Dottore. Updated April 25, 2022. Accessed April 28, 2022.

Keller, P. A., and D. R. Lehmann. "Designing Effective Health Communications: A Meta-analysis." *Journal of Public Policy and Marketing* 27, no. 2 (2008): 117–30.

Stuber, J., S. Galea, and B. G. Link. "Stigma and Smoking: The Consequences of Our Good Intentions." *Social Service Review* 83, no. 4 (2009): 585–609.

"Which Health Messages Work?" *ScienceDaily*, January 29, 2015. https://www.sciencedaily
.com/releases/2015/01/150129094345.htm. Accessed April 28, 2022.

"Workers Who Could Work at Home, Did Work at Home, and Were Paid for Work at Home,
by Selected Characteristics, Averages for the Period 2017–2018." US Bureau of Labor
Statistics. https://www.bls.gov/news.release/flex2.t01.htm. Updated September 24,
2019. Accessed April 28, 2022.

RESISTING THE ALLURE OF
MORAL GRANDSTANDING

We are living in an age of the visible moral gesture. It seems that all events of some note in our cultural or political life are accompanied by statements of support or opprobrium from anyone with a Twitter account. Social media has democratized the opportunity to weigh in. It allows us to instantly speak in support of, or against, causes we feel are worthy of attention, with hashtags amplifying our words.

These gestures are often made with the best intentions, and the sentiment they reflect—the wish to engage in the act of building a better world through praising the praiseworthy, or the converse—is admirable. There is no question that some of this making of social media statements has brought attention to important issues, elevating necessary conversations. But it also makes me wonder if our focus on these gestures is really helping to advance the cause of creating a better world. Could our outpouring of moral gestures on the occasion of, well, everything be less effective than we think? Could it even be a distraction from what we should be doing to shape a better future? Perhaps worse, could it encourage illiberalism in public health by causing us to think that if we make the right public gestures it doesn't matter what we substantively *do*, even if our actions undermine our liberal inheritance?

These questions raise the uncomfortable issue of moral grandstanding. By this term, originating in psychology, I mean acting and speaking in ways that project the appearance of morality not for the sake of issues themselves, but as a means of reaping the social benefits of being seen to be a good person. It is similar to a term many of us have heard: "virtue signaling." Such behavior has long been with us. History and literature are full of characters who have achieved status by broadcasting a virtue they may or may not actually possess. Moral grandstanding, and the tendency toward hypocrisy, is also warned against in some of the major religions, as in this passage from the Gospel of Matthew, a tenet of Christianity:

Be careful not to do your "acts of righteousness" before men, to be seen by them. If you do, you will have no reward from your Father in heaven.

So when you give to the needy, do not announce it with trumpets, as the hypocrites do in the synagogues and on the streets, to be honored by men. I tell you the truth, they have received their reward in full.

But when you give to the needy, do not let your left hand know what your right hand is doing, so that your giving may be in secret. Then your Father, who sees what is done in secret, will reward you.

And when you pray, do not be like the hypocrites, for they love to pray standing in the synagogues and on the street corners to be seen by men. I tell you the truth, they have received their reward in full.

But when you pray, go into your room, close the door and pray to your Father, who is unseen. Then your Father, who sees what is done in secret, will reward you. (Matthew 6:1–34, NIV)

Few of us can say we have not, at one time or another, indulged in moral grandstanding. With social media, moral grandstanding takes on a whole new prominence, because we can all perform for everyone to see, with instant affirmation (more followers, more likes). One could argue that it has become a form of recreation in recent years, as our technologies have made it easy to instantly weigh in on any issue. This has arguably tempted us away from more traditional forms of feedback, such as peer review, and toward the instant rush of social media feedback loops and the affirmation that comes with appearing virtuous to a supportive public. In our defense, perhaps, these technologies have made it challenging to do anything in private even when we wish to, so closely intertwined with our lives have they become. Speaking out at all, then, is often amplified by technology, as this technology becomes ever more synonymous with everyday speech.

Why am I raising the issue of moral grandstanding? After all, it may strike us as perhaps annoying, but not as something to take all that seriously. However, I suggest that it is indeed significant for efforts to build a healthy world. It has consequences not just for how we talk about health, but for our ability to pursue effective solutions to the problems we face. And it is central to the danger of illiberalism in public health. When we become accustomed to moral grandstanding, and to the applause and validation it can bring, we may find it harder to see where we have gone astray, even when we have traveled far along the path to illiberalism. For this reason, it is important to talk about the danger of moral grandstanding, toward supporting a liberal public health.

Given the proliferation of moral grandstanding in the age of social media, it seems worth asking two questions. Do we morally grandstand about health? And if so, how does this negatively affect our efforts toward a healthier world?

That we indeed do morally grandstand about health is, I think, clear. We have seen this in the morally tinged criticism of those who did not follow public health guidance during the pandemic and in the tendency, common on public health Twitter feeds, to weigh in on social and political issues using language that reflects undue confidence in our place on the right side of history. There is, of course, a fine line between moral grandstanding and providing needed moral clarity. I am not saying we should stop trying to provide the latter for fear of tipping into the former. However, if we are honest with ourselves, it's hard not to see how most of us, from time to time, succumb to the temptation of moral grandstanding, of voicing an opinion not just to clarify a debate, but for the social rewards of being seen to be right.

To the second question: Are there negative consequences to this behavior? I would say yes. First, moral grandstanding is a distraction. It takes work to organize, coordinate, and sustain symbolic actions, from promoting social media campaigns to coordinating public protest over an extended period. This leaves less energy to devote to the difficult and often quiet work of creating a social, economic, and political basis for better health. Moral grandstanding can also distract us from the reality that the line between good and bad does not run between groups but is in fact a line we all walk as individuals, with varying degrees of success. It's also noteworthy that the work it distracts us from is the work of a liberal public health. It is the work of engagement, of building consensus, of generating the science that supports our measures and of implementing these measures only once we have cultivated sufficient buy-in among the populations we serve. When we trade this for the immediate gratification of moral grandstanding, we turn our backs on the fundamentals of our field.

Second, moral grandstanding makes it possible to mistake posturing for genuine progress. When we confuse seeming to create change with actually creating it, we risk being content with the appearance of doing necessary work while leaving the work itself undone. This can set back our efforts to promote health while fooling us into thinking we have made progress and can therefore, perhaps, afford to pay less attention to the issues. It can even serve as cover for hypocrisy and unwillingness to see the changes we say we want.

Third, when we morally grandstand, we can make it difficult to attract people who might support our cause but be uncomfortable following our lead by loudly articulating their views. It takes time and patient work to change people's minds, and when it appears this change must be accompanied by bumper stickers, statements on social media, and other proclamations, it can sow doubts about advocating for it. In this way, such grandstanding can be more than merely annoying; it can actively dissuade people from joining worthy causes, undermining the momentum of these movements. For public health to be truly inclusive, its message should be maximally charismatic, able to attract buy-in from wide swaths of the population. If we morally grandstand, we risk undercutting this support, to the detriment of our movement.

Perhaps the most fundamental objection to moral grandstanding is that it runs counter to the humility necessary for building a healthier world. While humility can coexist with an ingrained sense of morality, it cannot coexist with moral grandstanding. Indeed, the case could well be made that morality itself is warped by moral grandstanding, as we find our attitudes subtly shaped by trying to garner praise. Even when we are justified in showing off a bit, there will come a time when we are in the wrong, and in anticipation of that day, we should exercise humility in the moment, keeping our focus on doing the best we can without broadcasting our efforts.

This is all, admittedly, perhaps easier said than done. The temptation of moral grandstanding is always present in our work, and it is impossible not to yield to it from time to time. There is, I realize with some irony, an element of grandstanding in even talking about grandstanding as I have done here. And at core, everyone who tries to articulate a better way of living and organizing society, which is the work of public health, risks moral grandstanding. However, it is precisely by accepting this reality that we open the door to the humility that can help ameliorate it. This humility can also help us in those times when the steps that are right for health are not the ones that are most popular in the moment. In order to *do* right, then, we must give up trying to always *seem* right in the eyes of others. We are then free to do what is necessary in pursuit of a healthier world.

SOURCES

Galea, S. "A Case against Moralism in Public Health." *Healthiest Goldfish* (blog), February 12, 2021. https://sandrogalea.substack.com/p/a-case-against-moralism-in-public. Accessed April 28, 2022.

Matthew 6:1–34, NIV. Accessed via Massachusetts Institute of Technology. https://web.mit
.edu/jywang/www/cef/Bible/NIV/NIV_Bible/MATT+6.html. Accessed April 28, 2022.

Resnick, B. "Moral Grandstanding Is Making an Argument Just to Boost Your Status. It's
Everywhere." *Vox*, November 27, 2019. https://www.vox.com/science-and-health
/2019/11/27/20983814/moral-grandstanding-psychology. Accessed April 28, 2022.

RESISTING OUR
SUBURBAN IMPULSES

Suburbs can be terrific places. I live in a suburb, and I can think of few better places to raise a happy, healthy family. Suburbs represent stability and the ascent of the middle class, a trend that has significantly broadened access to the material resources that support health. Indeed, when we speak about creating a world that generates health by expanding access to these resources, the ideal would be for everyone to enjoy the level of well-being reflected by suburban life.

But this is not yet the case—far from it. This unfairness is enforced by policies that benefit those with more at the expense of those with less. It is also enforced by habits of thought that allow us, even if we consider ourselves progressive-minded, to oppose measures that would share some of our advantages with others. These habits echo the presence of illiberalism in public health, as we find ourselves preaching virtues we don't always practice. Sadly, perhaps inevitably, there is a racial element to this, just as there is to the broader gap between the rich and the poor, and addressing this situation means speaking honestly about the full dynamics of the issue, including its intersection with race. I was struck by an article written in 2020 by former Minneapolis mayor Betsy Hodges, where she tackled this uncomfortable truth, saying, "White liberals, despite believing we are saying and doing the right things, have resisted the systemic changes our cities have needed for decades. We have mostly settled for illusions of change, like testing pilot programs and funding volunteer opportunities."

Such observations are, I think, bracing and necessary. It is easy to see how ideological opponents can block progressive change; it is perhaps more difficult to see how our own blind spots can stymie progress. These same blind spots can give cover to our turns toward illiberalism. It is worth examining the forces that shape our occasional hypocrisy around issues of core importance to health. The better we understand these forces in other contexts, the better we can understand them when they play a role in instigating the illiberalism we are all too capable of. In this chapter, then,

I will address the suburban impulses that can sweep those of us who are committed to the pursuit of justice off the path that leads to better health for all, and I will suggest ways we can resist these impulses so as to create a healthier world.

What do I mean by suburban impulses? Fundamentally, they are captured by an acronym NIMBY, "not in my backyard." NIMBYism is when people living in a community oppose measures that would support the public good in that community if these measures would in some real or imagined way encroach on their own convenience. A corollary is that this opposition can come from people who would support such measures as long as they happen somewhere else.

A classic example of NIMBYism occurs with affordable housing. Safe, affordable housing is a necessary condition for health, core to a progressive vision for a healthier world. Yet when the prospect of building affordable housing arises in communities, including those whose political composition is broadly left-leaning, pushback can emerge against building such units within their borders. This pushback can be prompted by concern over property values and over changes to the physical layout of the community, or it can indeed be fueled by animus toward the prospect of people of a different race or socioeconomic position moving into town.

This hypocrisy plays into the depiction of suburbs we often see in books, films, and television shows as places of artifice, in which a sunny exterior hides less appealing truths. Such fictionalized depictions can be quite dark; I have always preferred the more comedic framing of *The Truman Show*. The film depicts an idealized suburban life for its protagonist, Truman Burbank, who learns in the course of the story that his life is, in fact, an elaborately staged reality television show. While NIMBYism does not neatly match the premise of *The Truman Show*, both fact and fiction are linked by the phenomenon of communities appearing to be one way and then being revealed as another way.

Why does this matter to public health, and in particular to the vision of a liberal public health this book aims to support? Fundamentally, it matters on three levels. First, any action in the social or policy space that is motivated by wariness toward "the other," or by racism and hate, is bad for health. When these attitudes animate our thinking about the way we shape our communities, they undermine the capacity of these communities to be as healthy as they can be and further jeopardize the health of the vulnerable, who are already being excluded from the resources that generate health. Second, it entrenches the impulse that pulls us away from change, causing us to resist progress in favor of a status quo that does not distribute health equally. It is more than a failure of policy or compassion; it is a failure of imagination—the ability to picture a community that puts the good of all ahead of the fears and prejudices of some. Such an ability is at the heart of a liberal public health, sustained by centuries of progress informed by Enlightenment values. We can't exercise such imagination wearing NIMBY blinders. Third, NIMBYism reflects our human tendency to avoid doing what we know is best when doing so might curtail our own power, influence, or comfort. In this sense it echoes public health's occasional tendency to rank its own influence above the health of populations.

It is important to note, however, that our suburban impulses are not always characterized by the explicit rejection of measures that support the common good. Sometimes we are simply acting from a position of privilege to support measures we think are an unalloyed good for all, but that are actually onerous to those who live outside the picket fences of suburban comfort. We saw this during COVID, particularly in the conversation around lockdowns. Throughout the pandemic, those most able to navigate lockdowns were those living in safe, stable communities with plenty of space, material resources, access to electronic communications, and just enough distance from urban centers to justify an extended period of working from home: in short, those living in suburbs. And it was those lacking these advantages for whom extended lockdowns were particularly trying. Remote work was also much easier for those working in high-wage professions that support a suburban lifestyle and harder for those working in the sales and service jobs that tend to pay less. For example, data taken from the 2015 Canadian General Social Survey show how higher income can translate into more time working remotely, with those making $120,000 or more significantly likelier to work from home than those making less than $20,000. While these data predate COVID by a number of years, they are nevertheless instructive in showing the link between higher income and the capacity to work remotely.

This divide reflects how socioeconomic privilege shapes the means by which we have been able to navigate the pandemic. Those able to work from home were clearly in one place on the socioeconomic ladder and those less able to do so were on another. Yet this divide was not what most of us talked about when we discussed whether to embrace restrictive lockdowns.

This raises the question, Were those of us with a suburban mentality more willing to accept restrictive, at times borderline illiberal, COVID

rules because our relative comfort shielded us from their full consequences? It would be understandable for us to see the situation this way.
From this privileged perspective, there is relatively less downside to ongoing lockdowns than for someone who has fewer options for working from
home. This is not to say, of course, that working from home is entirely
without costs for those living in the suburbs, particularly for those with
children. But the cost-benefit analysis is radically different when seen from
both sides of the suburban/nonsuburban divide. This speaks to the power
of socioeconomic divides to inform a context in which illiberal thinking
(such as the embrace of draconian lockdowns imposed without public
buy-in or scientific support) can emerge, as I have discussed in previous
chapters.

How can we resist our suburban impulses, to make sure we are supporting policies that work for the good of all, not just for the privileged?
Core to doing so is the old saying, "To whom much is given, much is expected." We have a collective responsibility to ensure that the policies we
pursue support the health of as many people as possible. What is perhaps
ironic here is that many of those who have advocated for indefinite lockdowns likely thought this was precisely what they were doing—advocating
for the policy that was most conducive to the health of all. They could feel
this way because their socioeconomic advantages made it difficult for them
to see how it could be otherwise. This speaks to the importance of understanding the context that shapes health, so that we can recognize when
this context has positioned us to perhaps see the extent of our privilege
less clearly. We can then use our position to advocate for polices that truly
support the health of all.

SOURCES

Galea, S. "Housing and the Health of the Public." Boston University School of Public Health.
     https://www.bu.edu/sph/news/articles/2017/housing-and-the-health-of-the-public/.
     Published February 12, 2017. Accessed April 28, 2022.
Hodges, B. "As Mayor of Minneapolis, I Saw How White Liberals Block Change." *New York
     Times*, July 9, 2020. https://www.nytimes.com/2020/07/09/opinion/minneapolis
     -hodges-racism.html. Accessed April 28, 2022.
McIntosh, K., E. Moss, R. Nunn, and J. Shambaugh. "Examining the Black-White Wealth
     Gap." *Brookings*, February 27, 2020. https://www.brookings.edu/blog/up-front/2020
     /02/27/examining-the-black-white-wealth-gap/. Accessed April 28, 2022.   .
"NIMBY Definition and Meaning." Dictionary.com. https://www.dictionary.com/browse
     /nimby. Accessed April 28, 2022.

Petri, A. "Use the Quote Correctly or Not at All." *Washington Post*, April 16, 2015. https://www.washingtonpost.com/opinions/use-the-quote-correctly-or-not-at-all/2015/04/16/23bd81f2-e3ae-11e4-ae0f-f8c46aa8c3a4_story.html. Accessed April 28, 2022.

Tanguay, G. A., and U. Lachapelle. "Remote Work Worsens Inequality by Mostly Helping High-Income Earners." *Conversation*, May 10, 2020. https://theconversation.com/remote-work-worsens-inequality-by-mostly-helping-high-income-earners-136160. Accessed April 28, 2022.

CHECKING OUR BLIND SPOTS

The 1999 film *The Matrix* is about a man who discovers that the world as we know it is actually an elaborate simulation created by intelligent machines who use it to control humanity in the "real" world—a dystopian future where the machines have taken over. In the decades since its release, the premise of the film has become an established metaphor for realizing that the world as it is can sometimes be radically at odds with the world as we perceive it. As one close to home example of this, I can recall the moment when I realized that health is more than doctors and medicines; that health is, in fact, an emergent property of the world around us. I understood then that working to improve health means working to improve the world we live in, and that it is *that* world we should focus on.

Much of my career in public health has been an effort to make this very case—that a vision of health seeing only health care is incomplete; that when we talk about health we need to talk about far more than treatment alone. In the post-COVID era this strikes me as more important than ever. The nature of our pandemic experience was deeply, decisively shaped by the same factors that always shape health: politics, culture, the economy, the places where we live, work, and play, our social networks, and other structural forces that shape our world. Preventing the next pandemic means engaging with these forces to shape a healthier society. It means seeing health differently.

This book is in part a call to look at public health in a different light. It's a call to recognize that much of what we have accepted as normal in recent years is in fact not normal, that it is contrary to the animating principles of a liberal public health. Seeing this requires us to first look beyond the biases that blind us to reality—the reality of our field and, more broadly, of the world we are trying to make healthier.

If we can better understand our biases, perhaps better see what we are doing right and what we are doing wrong as a public health community, we can then work to correct our course where necessary, toward the aim of supporting a liberal public health.

To better understand bias, it is helpful to look at specific examples where bias has shaped our reasoning concerning health and prevented us from seeing the full picture. Let's first take the example of mental health and our engagement with mental illness. For a long time we didn't discuss mental health the way we discussed physical health—when we discussed it at all. Mental health—in particular, admitting to mental health struggles—was seen as taboo, a focus for stigma and shame. Happily this has begun to change. A number of high-profile people have opened up about mental health, from members of the British royal family to athletes like gymnast Simone Biles and tennis star Naomi Osaka. All this encourages conversations where mental health is more and more seen as on a par with physical health—as it should be.

But this evolving conversation, and its intersection with high-profile voices, has in my assessment been distorted by our individualist bias. In this case the individualist bias pushes us to think we are all equally vulnerable to poor mental health. The observation that prominent, wealthy persons struggle with mental illness further accentuates this point ("if they can have mental illness, so can anyone"). And while it is indeed true that anyone can suffer from poor mental health, and that we should have the compassion to recognize it, our individualist bias obscures the fact that mental health is subject to the same socioeconomic forces that create disparities in physical health, making certain populations more vulnerable than others. Money, housing, social networks, exposure to stressors—all these factors play a part in shaping mental health. Because access to assets like money and decent housing is more tenuous among the socioeconomically vulnerable, these populations are at greater risk of mental illness, particularly when crisis strikes.

This was well illustrated during COVID-19. At that time I was part of a research team that found depression rates among US adults tripled during the pandemic. We also found that lower income, less in savings, and greater exposure to stressors were linked with greater depression risk. Later our team published the first yearlong longitudinal study of depressive symptoms during COVID. The study was conducted on the same representative sample of US adults as the first study, having followed this group from spring 2020 to spring 2021. We found that, unlike the situation after other traumatic events, where depression tends to taper off in the long term, depression during COVID remained high. We also found that stressors such as housing, lack of child care, and job loss were all linked with greater depression one year into COVID.

In many ways these data confirm common sense in our thinking about mental health. Imagine, for example, that "Diana," who has long struggled to make ends meet, is working multiple low-wage jobs yet always falling behind. This burden, combined with the responsibility of caring for two children and the challenge of living in a poor, unsafe neighborhood with few friends or family nearby to help her, caused her to suffer from depression. Now imagine her facing these problems during the COVID pandemic. Imagine she lost one of her jobs and couldn't find a new one. Imagine her fearing for her children's safety and having to look after them at home every day during a year of school closures. In these circumstances it is no wonder she might find herself suffering from depression that is deeper, and more prolonged, than what is experienced by people with fewer difficulties in their lives.

When presented in these personal terms, it's easy to see how socioeconomic context shapes vulnerability to poor mental health. It's also easy to see how such context can be overlooked in our conversation about mental health. Because people like Diana have fewer assets and less financial and social capital, they also tend to have less clout in the halls of power and less representation in the national debate about the issues that matter most to their health. This strongly suggests that efforts to improve the health of all, consistent with our vision in public health, must first entail a moment when the scales fall from our eyes and we clearly see the full range of conditions that shape health, beyond a narrow focus on doctors and medicines. And it means overcoming the temptation to blame individuals for their poor health, as our bias toward individual behavior at the expense of context can cause us to do.

Our findings, reflected in Diana's story, suggest that vulnerability to poor mental health is deeply shaped by socioeconomic context. When it comes to improving mental health, therefore, recognizing that all of us are at risk of poor mental health is a necessary but insufficient step toward transformative change. When we recognize the ubiquity of poor mental health, we must try to address the conditions that leave certain populations disproportionately vulnerable to mental illness. This means it is imperative to engage with mental health at the level of the forces that shape these conditions, particularly at the political and economic levels that determine access to the assets that support health. Such steps require us to look beyond our bias toward investing in health care alone and to invest in the structural conditions that support health.

With this in mind, we can see how our bias against seeing the full picture of health might obstruct this engagement, complicating our efforts to address mental health. It would be easy to continue thinking that no population is any more or less vulnerable to mental illness than any other, and that the only factor shaping such vulnerability is individuals' internal mental state. Seeing the structure that truly underlies mental illness takes a willingness to look beyond what may seem obvious, to get at the roots of health. This means first acknowledging that we have biases and recognizing where they may have led us astray.

Mental health is just one area where we have allowed our biases to distort our vision. Another such area may be police violence, specifically violence against communities of color. Such violence demands accountability and reform, and it is entirely appropriate that, as a country and as a public health community, we should have a serious conversation on how to address this injustice. In doing so there is an understandable temptation to think the threat of police violence is so significant that we should consider abolishing policing entirely or, at the very least, should regard policing as a broadly negative influence on the well-being of communities of color. Public perceptions of the scope of the problem reflect an encouraging level of engagement with the issue, but they don't always reflect its true numerical scope. Research has found that over half of those identifying as "very liberal" estimated that one thousand or more unarmed Black men were killed by police in 2019. The actual number, while still far too high—any number would be—is much lower than the common perception. Some databases indicate that in 2019 there were between thirteen and twenty-seven cases, while other informed estimates suggest it may have been between sixty and one hundred, or perhaps a bit higher. While it is true that Black Americans are killed by police at a disproportionately higher rate than white Americans, it is also true that public perception does not always align with the actual numbers.

Given these attitudes toward policing, it is not surprising that many people have adopted maximalist positions toward police reform or abolition. One could make the case that this is to the good, that such advocacy is necessary given the intolerability of even one killing at the hands of police. But is there a blind spot to this discussion?

If there is, it likely concerns the role of policing in preventing violent crime, and the need for such prevention in many places where communities of color live. Black Americans are significantly likelier than whites to be homicide victims. In 2019, for example, 7,484 Black or African Americans died from homicide, compared with 5,787 whites. This challenge is reflected by the attitudes of Black Americans toward policing, with majorities in favor of keeping police in their communities. As of summer 2020, 61 percent of Black Americans said they wanted police presence in their area to remain the same, and 20 percent said they wanted police to spend more time in their area. It's important to note that these data coexist with other polling that shows widespread feeling among both Black and white Americans that Black populations are not treated as fairly as whites by the police and the criminal justice system. These data reflect a complicated reality. Black Americans do face injustice at the hands of police, and at the same time police play a central role in helping to protect Black communities.

However, the progressive discourse around policing does not always reflect this nuance, a blind spot that can have consequences for health. In 2020 murder rates soared in the United States, increasing by an average of 30 percent in thirty-four cities. In Minneapolis, for example, violence skyrocketed in the months following the killing of George Floyd, with violent crime rising by 21 percent. This includes a rise in homicides within the Black community, which continues to be disproportionately victimized by violence. At the same time, the city's police force saw an exodus of officers going on leave or retiring: at the end of October 2020, more than 130 were on extended leave. There is no single cause for this rise in violence, just as there is no single cause for poor health. The conditions of the pandemic, and resulting desperation and unemployment, likely played a significant role. But it would be naive to think attacks on policing in the wake of Floyd's killing did not also factor in. This speaks to the complexity of the issue of policing. Police sometimes abuse the communities they are meant to serve, but they also play a key, at times decisive, role in keeping them safe.

The upshot is that police violence is a complex, fluid issue with shades of gray and ample room for blind spots. The stakes of the conversation around policing are the lives and immediate safety of vulnerable populations. This makes it necessary to proceed carefully in this conversation, to work with compassion, good faith, and command of the data to try to get it right. It is also true that many of those in elite circles who engage with this conversation will not experience the consequences of getting it wrong. If our lack of nuance in talking about police violence creates a situation where more people of color are likely to fall victim to violent crime, it is doubtful that those of us privileged enough to work in the idea space, or the politicians who can access their own security detail, or the celebrity influencers weighing in on the debate will face these consequences. This suggests the importance of checking our blind spots, particularly when we engage from a position of privilege.

Bias is part of the human condition. We move through the world with an eye toward near-term survival and not necessarily considering the bigger picture of the forces that shape health. We tend to give priority to what seems most immediate and efficient over what addresses the deeper forces that shape our world. This is perhaps why we have been so vulnerable to illiberal thinking. Liberalism can be unwieldy and messy, and it is rarely as efficient as other forms of human organization, even as it safeguards the values that ensure long-term flourishing. Our bias toward immediate engagement with the urgent and the obvious has blinded us to the subtle and the long term. Just as we see physical health before we see mental health, we see what seems to help us in the moment before we see what supports a healthier future. This bias can cause us to embrace, for the sake of expediency, approaches that undermine the core tenets of our field, failing to support the future of a liberal public health. By recognizing our susceptibility to bias, I hope we can begin to reorient our vision toward seeing the forces that truly matter for health and embracing the liberal processes that are our best tool for engaging with them.

SOURCES

Alas, H. "2020 a 'Perfect Storm' for Homicide Surge." *US News and World Report*, February 4, 2021. https://www.usnews.com/news/national-news/articles/2021-02-04/2020-homicide-rates-spike-amid-pandemic-police-protests. Accessed June 9, 2022.

Bailey, H. "Minneapolis Violence Surges as Police Officers Leave Department in Droves." *Washington Post*, November 13, 2020. https://www.washingtonpost.com/national/minneapolis-police-shortage-violence-floyd/2020/11/12/642f741a-1a1d-11eb-befb-8864259bd2d8_story.html. Accessed June 9, 2022.

Blackwelder, C. "Prince Harry Says He and Meghan 'Chose to Put Our Mental Health 1st' When Exiting Royal Family." *Good Morning America*. https://www.goodmorningamerica.com/culture/story/prince-harry-meghan-chose-put-mental-health-1st-77823461. Published May 21, 2021. Accessed April 28, 2022.

Desilver, D., M. Lipka, and D. Fahmy. "10 Things We Know about Race and Policing in the U.S." Pew Research Center. https://www.pewresearch.org/fact-tank/2020/06/03/10-things-we-know-about-race-and-policing-in-the-u-s/. Published June 3, 2020. Accessed June 9, 2022.

Ettman, C. K., S. M. Abdalla, G. H. Cohen, L. Sampson, P. M. Vivier, and S. Galea. "Preva-
    lence of Depression Symptoms in US Adults before and during the COVID-19 Pandemic."
    JAMA Network Open 3, no. 9 (2020): e2019686.

Ettman, C. K., G. H. Cohen, S. M. Abdalla, L. Sampson, L. Trinquart, B. C. Castrucci,
    et al. "Persistent Depressive Symptoms during COVID-19: A National, Population-
    Representative, Longitudinal Study of U.S. Adults." *Lancet Regional Health* 5, no. 100091
    (2021): 1–12.

"Expanded Homicide Data Table 2." Uniform Crime Reporting (UCR) Program–FBI.
    https://ucr.fbi.gov/crime-in-the-u.s/2019/crime-in-the-u.s.-2019/tables/expanded
    -homicide-data-table-2.xls. Accessed June 9, 2022.

Galea, S. *Well: What We Need to Talk about When We Talk about Health*. Oxford: Oxford
    University Press, 2019.

Jany, L. "Minneapolis Violent Crimes Soared in 2020 amid Pandemic, Protests." *Star
    Tribune*, February 6, 2021. https://www.startribune.com/minneapolis-violent
    -crimes-soared-in-2020-amid-pandemic-protests/600019989/. Accessed June 9, 2022.

McCaffree, K., and A. Saide. "How Informed Are Americans about Race and Policing?"
    Skeptic Research Center, CUPES-007. 2021. https://www.skeptic.com/research-center
    /reports/Research-Report-CUPES-007.pdf. Accessed June 9, 2022.

McCarthy, N. "U.S. Police Shootings: Blacks Disproportionately Affected." Statista. https://
    www.statista.com/chart/21857/people-killed-in-police-shootings-in-the-us/. Published
    July 15, 2020. Accessed June 9, 2022.

Moran, B. "The Other End of the River." *Bostonia*, summer 2016. https://www.bu.edu/bos
    tonia/summer16/sandro-galea-public-health/. Accessed April 28, 2022.

Osaka, N. "Naomi Osaka: 'It's O.K. Not to Be O.K.'" *Time*, July 8, 2021. https://time.com
    /6077128/naomi-osaka-essay-tokyo-olympics/. Accessed April 28, 2022.

Predit, R. "First Year of Pandemic Saw Depression Rates Triple." *U.S. News and World
    Report*, October 5, 2021. https://www.usnews.com/news/health-news/articles/2021
    -10-05/first-year-of-pandemic-saw-depression-rates-triple. Accessed April 28, 2022.

Rosenfeld, R., T. Abt, and E. Lopez. *Pandemic, Social Unrest, and Crime in U.S. Cities: 2020
    Year-End Update*. Washington, DC: Council on Criminal Justice, 2021. https://build
    .neoninspire.com/counciloncj/wp-content/uploads/sites/96/2021/07/Year-End-Crime
    -Update_Designed.pdf. Accessed June 9, 2022.

Saad, L. "Black Americans Want Police to Retain Local Presence." Gallup. https://news
    .gallup.com/poll/316571/black-americans-police-retain-local-presence.aspx. Published
    August 5, 2020. Accessed June 9, 2022.

Silva, D. "'We're Human, Too': Simone Biles Highlights Importance of Mental Health in
    Olympics Withdrawal." *NBC News*, July 27, 2021. https://www.nbcnews.com/news
    /olympics/we-re-human-too-simone-biles-highlights-importance-mental-health
    -n1275224. Updated July 28, 2021. Accessed April 28, 2022.

Stellino, M. "Fact Check: Police Killed More Unarmed Black Men in 2019 Than Conserva-
    tive Activist Claimed." *USA Today*, June 23, 2020. https://www.usatoday.com/story
    /news/factcheck/2020/06/23/fact-check-how-many-unarmed-black-men-did-police
    -kill-2019/5322455002/. Accessed June 9, 2022.

Williams, B. "Homicides Go Unsolved as Killings in Minneapolis Rise." *MPR News*, Decem-
    ber 28, 2020. https://www.mprnews.org/story/2020/12/28/homicides-go-unsolved-as
    -killings-in-mpls-rise. Accessed June 9, 2022.

WE NEED TO TALK ABOUT CLASS

A liberal system—or any system—gains its legitimacy from its capacity to deliver for people. One of the best arguments for liberalism is its success in generating material resources in the parts of the world where it is ascendant. It is by no means perfect in this. Deep inequalities remain within liberal frameworks, and there is often unfairness within the system. But compared with where we were just a century ago, the average person has done far better than her forebears and has done so in a context that aims to maximize not just material well-being but freedom and civil equality in the public sphere. Yet there remain divides within liberalism that, if left unaddressed, could indeed threaten the integrity of our system. Perhaps the main dividing line is class—a test for both public health and liberalism. The divide between those with material resources and those with less is also a health divide. And some consider the very existence of such a divide within our liberal order to be evidence that our entire system is not worth keeping—an argument I reject. Within public health, class—defined along both social and economic lines—can create divides between our field and the populations we serve. Class is reflected in everything from the educational attainment of public health professionals to the elite institutions in which we often serve to the cultural and media spaces we inhabit. Class therefore is a proxy for many of the key challenges I have raised in this book, from media feedback loops to the power and influence we have enjoyed and perhaps have worked a bit too hard to preserve. The extent to which public health has become not just a field but a class is in large part the extent to which we have become attached to a perspective that does not serve us well in our work and can lead in illiberal directions. It is necessary, then, that we talk about class, to better understand the forces that pose a threat to the integrity of public health and, more broadly, to the health of populations.

My perspective on class is inextricably linked to my experience as an immigrant. One of the striking aspects of being an immigrant is the perspective it affords on one's adopted country: it can make obvious to the newcomer elements of the culture that native-born citizens might not see so clearly. As an immigrant to the United States, I found this true, just as an American likely would find on immigrating to my home country of Malta. I had not been here long before I realized something that is rarely acknowledged by those who grew up here but is quite clear to the immigrant: we do not often talk about class. This is particularly striking to the immigrant, because in so many countries class is among the defining features of a society. It is everywhere. In many places, sensitivity to class is so ingrained that it is possible to tell people's places in the social hierarchy before they even open their mouths. In America this consciousness is far less pronounced. Perhaps this reflects the egalitarian values enshrined in the country's founding premise that all are created equal. If this is the ideal we aspire to, it makes sense that we would downplay or overlook class.

Yet just because we don't talk about class doesn't mean it isn't a ubiquitous, fundamental determinant of health. In referring to class, I mean the socioeconomic status that informs a social hierarchy, with some people at the top and some at the bottom of the distribution of advantage. Given the foundational role of socioeconomic status in shaping health outcomes, it is not possible to avoid talking about the effects of class when talking about health, even while we are perhaps squeamish about calling this a conversation about class per se. Certainly other movements aspiring to reimagine social structures toward radical change have not shied away from this conversation. This is perhaps most famously so with the Marxist critique of the capitalist system, which has at its heart a vision of the perceived tension between those at the top of the socioeconomic hierarchy and those at the bottom. This reflects an effort to engage with the core drivers of inequity and suffering in society, with the aim of changing structures to engineer a better world. Indeed, Marx himself wrote, "To be radical is to grasp things by the root." His focus on class was an extension of this effort to address the roots of societal problems as he saw them. This focus strikes me as a necessary one in our engagement with the core drivers of health, even though many of Marx's conclusions remain vulnerable to criticism, to say nothing of the disastrous results of attempting to use his philosophies as the basis for running a state.

Fundamentally, health is about the conditions we live in; these conditions intersect with class in many ways. We are likelier to be healthy if we live in a nice house in a good neighborhood, if we attend good schools, if we have enough money in the bank to support us in times of crisis and

allow us access to goods, services, and leisure activities, if we have political, economic, and social clout. And the fact is, we are likelier to have all
these assets and more if we are upper class, or upper middle class, and we
are likelier to lack them if we fall closer to the bottom rung of the socioeconomic ladder.

Despite the importance of class in shaping the health of populations,
public health has been reluctant to address class directly. We tend to talk
around it, discussing its effects on health while rarely using the word itself.
This is perhaps because of the progressive, broadly left-leaning identity of
public health. Within this context, there can be a discomfort with class
consistent with a discomfort in left-leaning circles with the very idea of
socioeconomic hierarchy, to say nothing of the fact that we ourselves may
occupy its upper echelons. Acknowledging class means facing the ways
our society generates the unequal outcomes that can cause resentment,
conflict, and poor health. We have generally been much more comfortable
talking about identity than about the class structures our lives and health
intersect with. This echoes a lively debate that has been unfolding on the
left about whether to emphasize universalist language about class and economics or to continue to advance a more identity-focused argument when
making a case to voters.

It's worth noting that our hesitancy to talk about class is in some ways a
function of class itself. While we might not acknowledge class, the socioeconomic realities of our system are a daily presence in the lives of those
they disadvantage. These populations do not have the luxury of ignor-
ing the way the country is divided into haves and have-nots. When they
feel their concerns are being ignored by the ruling class, they may turn to
populist political movements that advance an illiberal approach to policy
and governing, which only exacerbates the class divides that have helped
bring about such movements. When they feel that we in public health are
to some extent part of this ruling class, they are less inclined to trust us
and more inclined to regard us with fear and hostility. They are likelier to
take this view when they see us acting illiberally.

How, then, can a liberal vision of public health address class, with the
aim of creating a world where class divides no longer pose problems for
health? Centrally, it can do this by creating a world where all can flourish. Creating such a world is primarily the work of politics, prompting
the question, What do we want from our political system? The answer,
it seems to me, amounts to three words: assets, opportunities, and dignity. Assets are the material resources that support health, whose lack or

abundance does so much to define and deepen class divides. Opportunities are chances to improve our station in life, to rise according to our abilities or be supported according to our need. Class divides are also opportunity divides, in which the rich have more and the less well-off have less. Working through politics, we can help expand the range of opportunities for all. We can do this from the bottom up by investing in a robust social safety net to support the most vulnerable, and from the top down, by curtailing unfair advantage for those who already have much. Finally, there is dignity. Class divides can be insidious in that they can rob those at the lower end of the hierarchy of their dignity, either through outright dehumanizing or through a lifetime of subtle snubs and reminders to "remember your place." While this may not be as explicit in the United States as in other countries, it is certainly a presence, undermining the dignity of many. Addressing class, then, means having a politics, and a culture, that supports dignity for everyone. We can achieve this right now. Although it can take time for policy solutions to be passed and implemented, nothing is stopping those in positions of leadership from shifting their emphasis from serving first and foremost the needs of the upper class to attending to the less well-off. Simply feeling listened to can do much to support the dignity of the often overlooked poor and working-class people.

Our engagement with class should also recognize the fundamental link between socioeconomic status and health. It is tempting to think we don't really need to talk about class in shaping a healthier world. All we need to do is provide quality health care to all and this will level the playing field on who gets to be healthy in our society. But while health care is important and should indeed be a human right, it is not enough, on its own, to close the health gap between classes. Health emerges from the world around us, and our experience of the world is indelibly shaped by class. Populations with poorer socioeconomic status have long had worse health, just as the advantages of wealth have long been a boon for health. For example, it remains a fact that the wealthiest men in the United States live an average of fifteen years longer than the poorest men, and the wealthiest women live an average of ten years longer than the poorest women.

This means we need an approach to class that proactively engages with socioeconomic status as an explicit means of improving health. Good health is a universal aspiration. During COVID-19 we learned that we *can* take dramatic steps as a society, and have difficult conversations, when we feel that health demands it. Our shared desire for health, then, can be a powerful tool to get us talking about class in the United States, perhaps encouraging a collective motivation to tackle class in a way it has not been seriously addressed over the centuries.

SOURCES

"Commonsense Solidarity: How a Working-Class Coalition Can Be Built, and Maintained." *Jacobin*, November 9, 2021. https://www.jacobinmag.com/2021/11/common-sense -solidarity-working-class-voting-report. Accessed April 28, 2022.

Galea, S. "A Populist Public Health." *Healthiest Goldfish* (blog), November 12, 2021. https:// sandrogalea.substack.com/p/a-populist-public-health. Accessed April 28, 2022.

———. "Who's Left?" *Healthiest Goldfish* (blog), March 19, 2021. https://sandrogalea .substack.com/p/whos-left. Accessed April 28, 2022.

Link, B. G., and J. Phelan. "Social Conditions as Fundamental Causes of Disease." *Journal of Health and Social Behavior*, 1995, special issue, 80–94.

Locke, J. *An Essay concerning Human Understanding*. Ed. K. Winkler and K. Marx. London: Hackett, 1996.

Reuell, P. "For Life Expectancy, Money Matters." *Harvard Gazette*, April 11, 2016. https:// news.harvard.edu/gazette/story/2016/04/for-life-expectancy-money-matters/. Accessed April 28, 2022.

PUBLIC HEALTH AND TRADITION

Public health is by nature forward looking. We aspire to a progressive vision of the future, one that supports health through a radical reimagining of the status quo. This goal calls on us to envision new ways of structuring our world, with an eye toward optimizing it for health. Our pursuit of this vision leads us to explore novel approaches to supporting health, to innovate, and to embrace new ways of thinking about the world and about living in it. Recall that many public health tools and interventions we now take for granted—like hand washing, public sanitation, and designing urban spaces with an eye toward health—were once new, and were even seen as radical. Their success speaks to the importance of a public health that is moving ever forward, eyes fixed on the possibilities of the future.

At the same time, a desire for progress can tempt us to sweep away all that came before. As I have written, a key danger in a liberal public health has been forgetting our roots as we have drifted away from the traditions of free speech, reasoned inquiry, and the pursuit of truth. This drift is understandable. In our efforts to discard what has been unproductive and unjust about the past, we can come to see even the positive elements of our inheritance as fundamentally compromised. Yet there is danger in forgetting our roots, throwing out the good with the bad. History provides many examples of how an overcorrection can lead to revolutionary excess and of the illiberalism that can attend such movements. This is of course not to compare a progressive public health to, say, the French Revolution. Yet we should look at our engagement with tradition to see that our zeal to improve on it doesn't at times give way to a zeal to dismiss it altogether, even when that means dismissing our liberal inheritance.

Having established that a vision of progress matters, we can then ask, Is it all that matters? Is a relentless focus on the future both necessary *and* sufficient for getting us to a healthier world? Such a focus is not, in fact, enough. For public health to be most effective, it should balance a focus on the future with a respect for—and willingness to learn from—what has served us well in the past. We should pay special attention to what has been handed down through the generations: tradition.

There are three key reasons tradition matters. First, innovation is rarely completely original and forward looking. More often it tends to resemble a patchwork quilt of ideas old and new. Consider music. The Beatles are widely considered one of the most original bands ever, creating songs that changed the craft of popular songwriting. Yet the band also drew on many existing musical traditions—from blues to jazz to music hall arrangements. These influences are close to the surface of the Beatles' music and were integral to what the band accomplished. Their work then became part of this musical tradition, influencing a range of later groups. The same goes for the uses of tradition in other areas, including health. We stand on the shoulders of giants, and if we are to uplift future generations, our efforts should start with respect for the traditions we have inherited—from religion to philosophy to cultural knowledge.

Second, when we engage with tradition, we maintain a connection to the best of the past, to the cultural richness that emerged from what came before. This includes the tradition of small-*l* liberalism that has done so much to support a better world through an embrace of freedom, human rights, and the legacy of the Enlightenment that informs many present-day goods, from our political system to the scientific method. This inheritance helps us advance a liberal public health by pursuing gradual reform through reason. The framework within which this pursuit unfolds—one of free and open debate, civility, respect for the individual, and the broader context of representative democracy and a rights-based social order—is itself a tradition, of which we are temporary stewards, and can help us create the better world we aim to see.

Third, respect for tradition supports the humility necessary for building a healthier world. It's tempting to think we know better than our forebears, that our science, technology, and moral sophistication put us miles ahead of them. But our forebears were people just like us, confronting many of the same issues. We should have the humility to recognize that those who came before us may have been attuned to certain truths that we in the modern age have missed. This is not to say we should embrace everything that has been passed down to us, but when tradition serves us well we should have the humility to acknowledge it, with gratitude.

This is not necessarily easy. Embracing tradition is in some ways counterintuitive. Often in public health, we find ourselves in a position of having to push back against an entrenched status quo that harms health and that may well be supported by destructive ideas embedded within tradition. A key example is hostility to the rights and dignity of LGBTQ individuals, a hostility that intersects with some of the oldest religious traditions in the world. Yet it is also worth noting that some of those same traditions have helped codify within societies compassion, concern for the marginalized, and a range of social norms that have done much to aid progress and support the advance of justice at critical points. In engaging with tradition, then, we need the sophistication to discern the good and the bad in what has been passed down to us, building on the good while rejecting the bad.

We see this reflected in our understanding of American history. America has committed great crimes—centrally, the injustice of slavery and genocide against indigenous populations. This history should be taught honestly, in full, even as we engage with the values and traditions that have come to us from our past. These traditions include religious liberty, freedom of speech and assembly, acknowledgment of the rights of ever-greater numbers of people, the triumphs of our art and culture, and our capacity to integrate a diverse range of nationalities and ethnic groups into a cohesive national project at a scale never before seen in human history, all while maintaining a standard of living that—for all the deep inequality remaining with us—is likewise unprecedented.

Striking a balance between appreciating the best of our tradition and acknowledging the often ghastly history it intersects with is a demanding, at times contentious, project. But it is one we must engage in. Throughout our history, the good in our liberal tradition has served as a lens showing us with ever-greater clarity how we are not living up to our ideals. Indeed, a key reason we can now have more nuanced conversations about justice, race, and health is long-standing awareness that we have fallen short of our founding values that say all are created equal. These values may have emerged in a compromised context, nested within the hypocrisies of those who first articulated them and a system that did indeed oppress and exploit. But just as gold is no less valuable for being found in the dirt, the all-too-human failings that characterized our country's founding and subsequent history do not negate the truth of America's core principles and their importance in shaping a better world. We should think critically about our traditions, question them, and never let them off easy. But we should also recognize the world-changing good they have done and acknowledge how necessary they remain in our present moment.

G. K. Chesterton once wrote about two types of reformer who encounter a fence blocking the road. The first, a "more modern" type, could not immediately see what the fence was for, so he argued that it should be torn down, since it was impeding progress. The second reformer considered that although the purpose of the fence was not immediately clear, it was likely built for a reason, so it was best to think deeply about what that reason might be before tearing the fence down. This speaks to both the importance of thinking about the uses and historical roots of tradition and of being aware of the temptation to reflexively do away with tradition without considering why it emerged in the first place and what role it still might play in shaping a better world. We need to balance respecting the uses of tradition with maintaining a forward-looking approach to health. Core to this is recognizing that we can look to the future only when we are supported by the achievements of the past. We should recognize these achievements, celebrate them, and build on their success.

SOURCES

Chesterton, G. K. Quotation. Goodreads. https://www.goodreads.com/quotes/833466-in -the-matter-of-reforming-things-as-distinct-from-deforming. Accessed April 28, 2022.

MY BIAS IN FAVOR OF LIVING

In science it is customary for researchers to disclose any potential bias as part of publishing their work. With this in mind, I will disclose my own bias, which has relevance for how I see the world and how I write about it. My bias is this: If presented with a choice between, on one hand, absolute safety at the cost of the interactions and experiences that make life worth living and, on the other, having these experiences with the understanding that they entailed some risk, I would choose the latter.

This matters because the way we engage with risk shapes how far we are willing to go to mitigate it. Often, for example, illiberal political movements arise because a population believes it is at risk. Decisions to set aside liberal tenets like free speech, freedom of assembly, and the rule of law are often framed as emergency measures embraced in response to risk. When we believe we are threatened, we are likelier to do whatever it seems will end the threat, even if this means dismissing basic civic principles. The temptation to do so is arguably even greater in light of public health's increasing unwillingness to engage with trade-offs, making us more apt to accept more zero-sum solutions.

My bias in favor of living, then, probably informs my concern over the illiberalism that public health can embrace in pursuit of an unrealistic ideal of total safety—such as its goal in some places of zero COVID. In some ways my bias may also be a product of my being an immigrant, one who has—like many immigrants—worked to construct a life in a new country, often in the face of uncertainty and risk. Although my journey from Malta to Canada to the United States has been far less difficult than the journey of many other immigrants, I nevertheless know what it is like to experience the challenges that are ever present in an immigrant's life. I also know what it is to choose to take on such challenges in search of a better life, to willingly accept uncertainty and risk because moving forward seems to demand it. All this background shapes my perspective on the steps we took for a feeling of greater security during COVID-19. It also helps clarify for me why we may turn toward illiberalism. We have restricted certain behaviors because they make us feel unsafe; we have discouraged certain conversations because they make us uncomfortable; we have aligned ourselves with one political party because we feel threatened by the other. All this speaks to a discomfort with uncertainty and risk that is so deep it makes us capable of neglecting our core principles.

Learning to live with uncertainty, then, is core to building a healthier relationship with risk, one that can inform a liberal public health. When we come to terms with uncertainty we are that much closer to realizing that life always entails some measure of risk, and that the challenge is to coexist with it rather than seeking to eliminate it through illiberal means.

As a result of my bias toward living, I found myself unable to dismiss concerns over the harmful effects of some COVID measures, even as I fully accepted the necessity of these measures in the face of a historic crisis. To be clear, the restrictions we embraced—from lockdowns to masking to distancing—were, on balance, the correct approach to the problem, if at times imperfectly applied. It's possible to acknowledge this while also acknowledging the cost they entailed. We accepted this cost because the alternative was clearly worse. We then reached a stage of the pandemic where this was no longer so clear. It was a liminal space, between where we had been for much of the pandemic and the full reopening of society. Within this space, we saw calls to maintain strict vigilance, even as vaccinations increased. Among demographic groups where vaccination was more or less complete—for example, older adults living in nursing homes—we remained hesitant to reopen society, even as the science supported the safety and efficacy of vaccines. The difference between the beginning of the pandemic and its later stage was that toward the end we had much more information, and therefore our risk calculus should have changed. We knew with more precision how the virus spread and who was at greatest risk. We also knew about the broader costs that mitigation efforts placed on society, ranging from mental illness to unequal economic loss to increases in substance misuse to reduction in non-COVID-related research.

This speaks to a broader problem when it comes to balancing risk. We are quick to identify risk, but we are slow to recognize how far we've come in mitigating it. We hesitate to trust our own success—whether our success in vaccine development or, more broadly, the progress we've made over the past century in creating a healthier world.

And we have indeed made progress. In many respects we live in a world that is better, healthier, than ever before. Global poverty has plummeted, maternal mortality is declining, and living standards have improved. The world is also less violent overall. This is not to say we don't still have problems—we do indeed. Yet we are sometimes liable to overemphasize the risks we face, or to emphasize the wrong risks, based on a lack of perspective about where we are relative to where we were. During COVID this tendency arguably manifested as the impulse to continue embracing lockdowns and restrictions even as the data and the reality of vaccines supported a return to a more open status quo.

What, then, did it mean to reopen, in a world where risk is ever present? First, it meant weighing liberties versus restrictions differently, not as a zero-sum proposition, but as an effort to strike a balance between living freely and taking prudent steps to safeguard health. Choices about health are complex and require trade-offs. We give a little liberty to get a little safety, and to give a little is not to give all (despite what many opponents of public health measures seem to think). Nor is it nothing to ask populations to sacrifice some freedom in the name of health (despite what many advocates of indefinite lockdowns seem to think). At the same time, we should be wary of tipping too far toward a pursuit of total safety at the expense of the openness that is the foundation of liberalism. Accepting that total safety is impossible, we should mistrust any approach that suggests it is achievable, particularly when that approach entails a turn toward illiberalism. We need to find a balance between safety and uncertainty, and part of that balance is accepting the risk that comes with living a life.

Second, it is important to give priority to what is good for the next generation. This was particularly relevant when children faced disruptions to their education as a consequence of COVID restrictions. The question of whether to open schools during the pandemic was, at core, a matter of sacrificing students' long-term capacity to live healthy lives in the interest of mitigating disease in the near term. Education shapes our ability to live healthy, fulfilling lives, and this is particularly true of the education we receive in our earliest years. The lack of nuance in our conversation about lockdowns, I would argue, consistently failed students, particularly younger students, as our willingness to pursue a sense of safety at all costs pushed aside the broader considerations that enable living a healthy life. This reflects a failure to give priority to the next generation in our thinking about health. It is also worth noting that health, in the long term, flourishes in a liberal context. Trading liberalism for the perception of safety may seem like a reasonable exchange in the short term, yet its long-term effect is a less healthy world. Investing in the next generation means investing in a liberal public health.

While these suggestions may reflect my personal bias, they also, I hope, constitute a useful approach to addressing the problems of the moment. Our engagement with risk shapes our engagement with liberalism. When our relation to risk is healthy, proportionate, we are better positioned to support a liberal public health that does not pursue its mission at the expense of the openness that makes life meaningful. Such a public health depends in part on being able to tolerate some level of uncertainty in our engagement with the world. Once we can do so, we can learn, whenever possible, to err on the side of living as we work to safeguard health.

SOURCES

"Disclosure of Potential Bias." Annual Reviews. https://www.annualreviews.org/page/authors/author-instructions/submitting/disclosure. Accessed April 28, 2022.

Galea, S. "Vaccines Can Give Older Adults Their Lives Back—We Should Let Them." *Toronto Star*, March 24, 2021. https://www.thestar.com/opinion/contributors/2021/03/24/vaccines-can-give-older-adults-their-lives-back-we-should-let-them.html. Accessed April 28, 2022.

Galea, S., R. M. Merchant, and N. Lurie. "The Mental Health Consequences of COVID-19 and Physical Distancing: The Need for Prevention and Early Intervention." *JAMA Internal Medicine* 180, no. 6 (2020): 817–18.

Giustini, A. J., A. R. Schroeder, and D. M. Axelrod. "Trends in Views of Articles Published in 3 Leading Medical Journals during the COVID-19 Pandemic." *JAMA Network Open* 4, no. 4 (2021): e216459.

Karageorge, E. X. "COVID-19 Recession Is Tougher on Women." US Bureau of Labor Statistics Monthly Labor Review. https://www.bls.gov/opub/mlr/2020/beyond-bls/covid-19-recession-is-tougher-on-women.htm. Published September 2020. Accessed April 28, 2022.

Maani, N., and S. Galea. "Science and Society Are Failing Children in the COVID Era." *Scientific American*, March 3, 2021. https://www.scientificamerican.com/article/science-and-society-are-failing-children-in-the-covid-era/. Accessed April 28, 2022.

"Overdose Deaths Accelerating during COVID-19." Centers for Disease Control and Prevention. https://www.cdc.gov/media/releases/2020/p1218-overdose-deaths-covid-19.html. Accessed April 28, 2022.

Porter, C. "Elderly, Vaccinated and Still Lonely and Locked Inside." *New York Times*, March 9, 2021. https://www.nytimes.com/2021/03/09/world/canada/canada-nursing-home-vaccine.html. Updated August 12, 2021. Accessed April 28, 2022.

Roser, M. "Measurement Matters–the Decline of Maternal Mortality." Our World in Data. https://ourworldindata.org/measurement-matters-the-decline-of-maternal-mortality. Published October 25, 2017. Accessed April 28, 2022.

————. "The Short History of Global Living Conditions and Why It Matters That We Know It." Our World in Data. https://ourworldindata.org/a-history-of-global-living-conditions -in-5-charts. Accessed April 28, 2022.

Roser, M., and E. Ortiz-Ospina. "Global Extreme Poverty." Our World in Data. https://our worldindata.org/extreme-poverty. Accessed April 28, 2022.

"Study Settles the Score on Whether the Modern World Is Less Violent." *ScienceDaily*, June 16, 2020. https://www.sciencedaily.com/releases/2020/06/200616113913.htm. Accessed April 28, 2022.

Hopes

Advancing a liberal vision for public health is at core a hopeful project. And despite the challenges of the present moment, there is indeed much cause for hope.

MERCY AND OUR
PRESENT MOMENT

In *The Merchant of Venice* William Shakespeare created a character who is entirely justified in seeking revenge. Shylock, a Jewish moneylender, has lived his life as the subject of constant anti-Semitic attacks, one of his main antagonists being Antonio, the merchant of the play's title. Antonio has called Shylock terrible names, assaulted him, and spit on him. So when Antonio defaults on a loan from Shylock, one for which the merchant offered a pound of his own flesh as security, Shylock is eager to collect. The audience—having witnessed the many injustices Shylock has suffered throughout the play—can find it hard to blame him. Yet something unexpected happens in the famous scene when Shylock demands what he is owed. It is there that Portia, a beautiful and intelligent heiress, begs Shylock to consider mercy:

> The quality of mercy is not strain'd,
> It droppeth as the gentle rain from heaven
> Upon the place beneath: it is twice blest;
> It blesseth him that gives and him that takes:
> 'Tis mightiest in the mightiest: it becomes
> The throned monarch better than his crown;
> His sceptre shows the force of temporal power,
> The attribute to awe and majesty,
> Wherein doth sit the dread and fear of kings;
> But mercy is above this sceptred sway;
> It is enthroned in the hearts of kings,
> It is an attribute to God himself;
> And earthly power doth then show likest God's
> When mercy seasons justice.

These words in defense of mercy complicate the scene of would-be vengeance. As anyone familiar with *The Merchant of Venice* knows, Shylock is justified in his anger. The play is rife with examples of anti-Semitism, including Shylock's eventual fate (he is ultimately thwarted in his pursuit of revenge and forced to convert to Christianity). This anti-Semitism should be deeply troubling to all readers and playgoers today, especially given the events of the past century and the recent resurfacing of anti-Semitic animus in the United States and globally. Yet despite—and perhaps because of—the context of Shylock's justified anger, mercy's appeal still resonates. It is an appeal worth thinking about in our current situation, and particularly in the context of health.

Indeed, much of present-day illiberalism reflects a spirit of condemnation and a lack of any consideration of the value of mercy. This is particularly evident in recent controversies over speech, in which discussing a taboo topic, or using ill-considered language, becomes grounds not just for strong disagreement from one's peers or reasoned engagement with what was said, but for firing and even informal professional blacklists. It is true, of course, that there are many ways one can say or do something that would warrant a strong response, even loss of a position. This could be said to be justice. But when mercy no longer seasons justice, we run the risk of illiberalism creeping into our engagement with each other and the ideas we work with. What's more, the rise of media feedback loops has made it easier to avoid interacting with those we disagree with, creating an environment where we can feel they are uniquely bad, even evil, and not worthy of mercy. Thus it is important that we think about mercy, its place in public health, and its role as a mitigating factor against illiberal excess.

It's worth noting that the tendency to dismiss mercy can emerge from an understandable, even laudable, impulse: anger over injustice. One of our core tasks in public health is to address injustices experienced by marginalized groups. These injustices are shaped by the same societal pathologies that birthed Shylock's misery and desire for vengeance. Scholarship in the area has given us a detailed, excruciating account of exactly how forces like racism, xenophobia, economic inequality, and the marginalizing of LGBTQ populations harm health. We know how many sicken and die needlessly owing to these forces. One of the most affecting moments of my career was when I worked on quantifying excess deaths attributable to social factors in the United States in the year 2000. We found that 245,000 deaths were attributable to education deficits, 176,000 to racial segregation, 162,000 to low social support, 133,000 to individual-level poverty, 119,000 to income inequality, and 39,000 to area-level poverty. Such findings are not just cause for sadness, they are cause for anger. This anger deepens when we consider how the brunt of poor health has long been borne by certain groups as a consequence of socioeconomic marginalizing. This can spark an urge to dismantle anything that could support such a broken status quo. Any system, political faction, or even person who seems to stand in the way of fixing this injustice becomes not merely an obstacle but an enemy, not something that is mistaken, but something that means harm.

This is how anger makes us think. Or, rather, how anger makes us feel. This feeling has arguably become the animating force behind the public debate in recent years. For a long time, both sides of the cultural and political divide in the United States could claim their project was essentially reformist. From the Great Society to the Reagan Revolution, the central, stated motivation of those looking to change the world through politics was to work within systems to shape a better world. This work could get combative at times, but an effort was made to maintain at least the appearance of working toward reform.

This is no longer the case. We now find ourselves navigating a political and cultural space in which the central goal is to a large extent punitive, calling not for mere progress but for a repudiation of all that has come before, to balance the scales. These feelings are understandable, and deeply human. When faced with injustice, our impulse is, reasonably perhaps, to hunker down, to attack when we can, to regain the upper hand, even through illiberal means.

But is this right?

On a personal level there is a case to be made that, in extending mercy, we serve our own well-being by letting go of the anger and grudges that can imprison us. The desire for revenge, even the fervent desire for what we would call justice, can be accompanied by that most corrosive of emotions: resentment. And to resent someone is, as the saying goes, like taking poison and expecting the other person to die. On a societal level, history provides many examples of how collectivized resentment can lead to terrible abuses when one group holds another accountable for past wrongs—real or imagined—and exacts a high price. The societal costs can include war, genocide, and cycles of revenge passed down through the generations. Resentment can build to these destructive climaxes or it can remain internalized, eating away at ourselves. What matters more than the scale of these outcomes is their shared source: an unwillingness to set aside anger and embrace mercy.

When we choose mercy, we immediately broaden our capacity to build a healthier world. We do this by accessing the compassion that is a companion to mercy and a necessary condition for health. I have often written and spoken about how compassion is fundamental to seeing clearly the conditions that create poor health and motivating us to change them. One of my favorite examples of this is the story of Equal Justice Initiative founder Bryan Stevenson, told in his memoir *Just Mercy: A Story of Justice and Redemption.* Much of the book centers on his work as a lawyer trying to overturn the conviction of a man on Death Row. Work to remove the stain on the soul of the country that is capital punishment would not be possible without the mercy that allows us to set aside our initial impulse to condemn people who may well have committed terrible acts. Walter McMillian, the man Stevenson helped, was wrongfully convicted, but this is to some extent immaterial where mercy is concerned. As seen with Shylock, the condemnation that mercy can temper is as often as not legitimate. That is why mercy is so powerful, and so necessary for stirring compassion. Stevenson's mercy birthed a compassion that led him to address the broader challenge of mass incarceration in the United States and the injustices that shape it. Who knows what new vistas compassion might bring into view for us once mercy helps clear away the resentments that can cloud our vision?

Finally, mercy links to the fundamental goal of public health: our aim is to create a healthier world so that all can live up to their full human potential, to flourish and to thrive. This suggests that we have an imperative to make sure everyone has access to a world free from preventable harm, so that everyone can be maximally healthy. Implicit in this is that we do not take actions that perpetuate cycles of anger, retribution, and hate. This does not mean denying the validity of anger and the many ways it can be justified, even be necessary. It means acknowledging anger while understanding that we live in the present, in a complex, messy, very human world. In such a world, the effects of anger simply cannot be allowed to unfold indefinitely, in all directions, if we are to make the world a place where we can all be healthy. Ultimately, mercy not only is the right course to take, it is the only course that will keep us from societal fracture, by bridging divides and ending the cycles of hate that have already done much harm.

SOURCES

Galea, S. "Compassion in a Time of COVID-19." *Lancet* 395, no. 10241 (2020): 1897–98.
———. "TEDMED: How Health Is Threatened by Hate" (video). YouTube. https://www.you tube.com/watch?v=WqwNUC34Tkw. Published April 29, 2020. Accessed April 28, 2022.

———. *Well: What We Need to Talk About When We Talk About Health*. Oxford: Oxford University Press, 2019.

Galea, S., M. Tracy, K. J. Hoggatt, C. Dimaggio, and A. Karpati. "Estimated Deaths Attributable to Social Factors in the United States." *American Journal of Public Health* 101, no. 8 (2011): 1456–65.

"Home." Equal Justice Initiative. https://eji.org. Accessed April 28, 2022.

"Just Mercy (book)." Wikipedia. https://en.wikipedia.org/wiki/Just_Mercy_(book). Updated March 25, 2022. Accessed April 28, 2022.

"The Merchant of Venice: Antonio." SparkNotes. https://www.sparknotes.com/shakespeare/merchant/character/antonio/. Accessed April 28, 2022.

"The Merchant of Venice: No Fear Translation." SparkNotes. https://www.sparknotes.com/nofear/shakespeare/merchant/. Accessed April 28, 2022.

"Resentment Is Like Taking Poison and Waiting for the Other Person To Die." Quote Investigator. https://quoteinvestigator.com/2017/08/19/resentment/. Published August 19, 2017. Accessed April 28, 2022.

Shakespeare, William. *The Merchant of Venice* (entire play). Massachusetts Institute of Technology: The Complete Works of William Shakespeare. http://shakespeare.mit.edu/merchant/full.html. Accessed April 28, 2022.

A CASE FOR GOOD
FAITH ARGUMENT

A healthy world is a world founded on good ideas, and good ideas are established through open, rigorous, even heated debate. Yet such debate is not always seen in our public discourse. Polarization has characterized a public conversation that does not always support a healthier world. Conducting better public debate entails trading the cynicism that often permeates bad faith arguments for the healthy skepticism that informs the generative conflict of ideas that truly advances progress. Good faith debate is also a hallmark of the liberal framework that supports a healthy exchange of ideas. Assuming good faith allows us to examine ideas based on their merits rather than on our personal feelings toward the individuals we engage with. It also helps us break out of the media feedback loops and hyperpartisanship that undermine a liberal vision of public health. A case for good faith argument, then, is a case for maintaining a critical norm that sustains such a vision.

Now is indeed the time for a revival of good faith debate. Polarization, informed by political divides, has come to characterize much of the public conversation. The time of COVID-19 was no exception—if anything, it intensified the division we have seen. It didn't take long after a novel coronavirus emerged for the existential stakes of the political debate to migrate to conversations about masking, lockdowns, social distancing, the origins of the virus itself, the means of treating the disease, and eventually vaccines.

These divides did much to undermine our response to the pandemic, just as they added dysfunction to our political process and frayed the social fabric. Having said this, let me add that I don't regard emotional, deeply felt debate as a uniformly negative influence. I have long argued for the importance of diverse perspectives and for creating space to air and debate these perspectives, even when such debates are uncomfortable and contentious. This discourse, when it is conducted with civility and respect, unfolding in a liberal framework, is necessary for advancing the ideas that support a healthier world and, ultimately, a culture and politics capable of meeting the needs of the moment.

There is, of course, a seeming inconsistency in what I have just said. How can I say divisions have undermined our COVID response—and, by implication, our broader approach to health—while also arguing that we need vigorous, even contentious, debate? I found myself inspired on this by reading what Supreme Court Justice Clarence Thomas wrote about his interactions with the late Justice Ruth Bader Ginsburg: "Justice Ginsburg and I often disagreed, but at no time during our long tenure together were we disagreeable with each other. She placed a premium on civility and respect."

If Justice Thomas and Justice Ginsburg, who disagreed with each other's views on the court most of the time, could argue for decades with civility and respect, so can we all. The key to this, I venture, lies in a central characteristic of any conversation where opposing views are presented, one that determines whether the conversation is constructive. That characteristic is the presence, or the lack, of good faith. By good faith I mean a spirit that puts forward ideas that are thoughtfully considered, with the goal of advancing a better world. Good faith arguments are presented in a way that respects the other position, with an eye toward learning and compromise, not zero-sum domination. This is in contrast to ideas advanced solely to support one's political "team," to gain advantage over one's perceived opponents, or simply to generate attention. Good faith arguments, then, are undermined by partisan commitments of the type we sometimes saw public health make during the pandemic. This reflects the link between good faith arguments and a liberal public health, one that places the reasoned pursuit of truth above any political bias.

The alternative to good faith arguments is a conversation characterized by bad faith refusal to accept that others may have good intentions in the case they are making. These arguments can be used to sow doubt about conclusions that are, in fact, scientifically sound. This is the case, for example, with arguments that tobacco is safe or that climate change is not real, two positions that are not supported by science but are strongly backed by financial and partisan incentives.

When ideas are presented in good faith, it is possible for a debate to become heated and still support progress. When they are not, then even ideas that are good in themselves are in a far weaker position for creating a better world. Indeed, presenting good ideas in bad faith can taint these ideas for years to come, robbing the public debate of arguments that might otherwise have been beneficial.

The Trump era was an effective test of this. I don't think it is partisan to say that former president Trump made many statements in bad faith. His overarching concern was to defeat his political opponents, and he often seemed to adopt positions solely for this purpose. This is not to say that Trump was the only purveyor of bad faith in the recent past. Perhaps in reaction, or perhaps illuminating more fundamental human truths, we saw bad faith arguments at every level of public discourse. During COVID there was no shortage of such arguments, as elements of our pandemic response were co-opted by partisans with all sorts of motivations. This is, I would stress, categorically different from robust, good faith debates aimed at achieving best practices to help us navigate a difficult moment. All this helped inform the illiberalism that emerged both within public health and in the broader political and social sphere. Indeed, the time of COVID helped clarify why it is necessary to differentiate between arguments made in good faith or in bad faith, as a means of advancing a liberal conversation that genuinely supports a healthier world.

How can we determine whether an argument is made in good faith or in bad faith? To my thinking there are two ways. The first way is rooted in a realistic view of human motivations. We can better understand the spirit in which the argument is being presented through a clear-eyed analysis of the incentive structure supporting it. For example, there are people and organizations whose job is to present the news from a sharply partisan perspective. Fundamentally this means that their business model depends not on the triumph of the best ideas, but on the ongoing slow burn of partisanship in our society. They may seem to want their ideas to win out, but if they did, the argument would be over, hurting their bottom line. So the continuation of rancorous debate will always be their core priority, even at the expense of the natural progression of ideas. It's not hard to see how such an incentive structure can corrupt the presentation of even the best ideas, creating a structural barrier to good faith debate. It's easy to see why, for example, much bad faith arguing happens on social media, where the incentive is to get likes and views, which accrue to any form of heated argument regardless of how reasoned (or not) it may be. This is a recipe for an illiberal public debate. Of course this does not mean everyone working within such an incentive structure is consciously acting in bad faith, only that the foundations of their endeavor make it hard to resist this counter-productive tendency. Although calling attention to these incentives may seem cynical when so much of our public debate is underwritten by these forces, to look away is to miss something fundamental about the nature of this conversation.

Yet it is not so much cynicism that helps us see the incentive structures that support bad faith; rather, it is skepticism. Indeed, it is cynicism that tends to *produce* so much bad faith in our society. Skepticism, on the other hand, is rooted in the tradition of scientific inquiry, in the empiricism that evaluates theories and ideas for their truth and general utility, not for their usefulness to a given ideology or partisan goal. As a way of neutralizing bad faith, skepticism could well be described as "doubting in good faith." It is through a healthy skepticism that we can detect the presence not just of bad faith but of bad arguments. This discovery opens the door to a robust, liberal process of debate and inquiry motivated purely by a search for the truth, the truth being a necessary condition for the best practices that support a healthier world. Skepticism frustrates the rush to judgment that so often accompanies bad faith arguments; it forces us to slow down, weigh evidence, and consider the broader context. This can counteract the tendency to reach a consensus too hastily, an error we saw not just during COVID, but with earlier health threats such as the Zika virus. As with COVID, the emergence of Zika presented us with many unknowns— about its origin, its effects, and how to best prevent it. This state of not knowing led to a rush to engage with this disease using approaches that had worked with past contagions like Ebola, even when this proved to be an uneasy mismatch. Had we paused to apply an appropriate skepticism to our efforts, we might well have avoided some of the blind alleys we found ourselves in.

Implicit in both these suggestions is the importance of balance. It is possible, and somewhat ironic, that both skepticism and a realistic awareness of incentive structures can themselves be used in bad faith, to discredit ideas we do not like. It's not uncommon, for example, to hear arguments opposed not on their merits, but owing to the occupation or identity of the person making them. Likewise, it is possible for healthy skepticism to curdle into a dogmatic unwillingness to accept new information or emerging paradigm shifts, however much they are based on solid empirical analysis. Both these perspectives, then, should be used judiciously, in good faith, to advance understanding.

It's worth asking, What might our pandemic experience have been like had it been informed more by good faith and healthy skepticism than by cynical put-downs and zero-sum partisanship? Given the power of the latter to narrow our idea space and limit our capacity to collaborate on solutions, it is likely that a more constructive engagement would have produced a better response to COVID. Working in good faith might have moved our conversation past scoring political points to support a nimbler, more data-informed coordination of best practices in the face of the pandemic.

Perhaps I'm naive in thinking we can set aside our tendency to engage with each other in bad faith. But the COVID crisis has shown what can happen when our arguments are shaped too much by cynicism and motivations that have little to do with creating a healthier world. Given that COVID could well be followed by a far more dangerous pandemic, we no longer have the luxury of being swayed by our worst motivations. We need to engage in good faith with the challenges we face if we are to shape a future that is healthier than our past.

SOURCES

Annas, G., S. Galea, and D. Thea. "Zika Virus Is Not Ebola." *Boston Globe*, February 1, 2016. https://www.bostonglobe.com/opinion/2016/02/01/zika-virus-not-ebola/gbBZA18IL kLcLK2VNM7XfM/story.html. Accessed April 28, 2022.

"Clarence Thomas Fondly Remembers 'Rapid' RBG." *Politico*, April 20, 2021. https://www .politico.com/news/2021/05/20/ruth-bader-ginsburg-clarence-thomas-489782. Accessed April 28, 2022.

Galea, S. "Health and the Opportunity to Freely Think." *Healthiest Goldfish* (blog), April 2, 2021. https://sandrogalea.substack.com/p/health-and-the-opportunity-to-freely. Accessed April 28, 2022.

———. "The False Choice between Diversity, Inclusion, and the Pursuit of Excellence." *Healthiest Goldfish* (blog), May 15, 2021. https://sandrogalea.substack.com/p/the-false -choice-between-diversity. Accessed April 28, 2022.

"Merchants of Doubt." Wikipedia. https://en.wikipedia.org/wiki/Merchants_of_Doubt. Accessed April 28, 2022.

"ONE DOES HAVE JOYS"

Public health is fundamentally about trying to create a world that is healthier, and thus better. In doing this work we must at times comment, a priori, on how we are falling short on generating health. This can make a discipline that is all about health seem chiefly concerned with sickness, since we so often discuss its causes and its consequences. This conversation is necessary for the work of public health. But it is worth asking, Can this keep our attention fixed on problems at the expense of the more positive aspects of health—all the ways health can enable a happy life? The question may seem frivolous compared with this book's broader argument about addressing illiberalism in public health. However, our choice to emphasize either positive or negative aspects of health shapes our pursuit of a healthier world. If we lean into the negative, we are likelier to cultivate an engagement with our work that is likewise negative, mistrustful. When this happens it is not hard to see how, faced with a public that does not particularly like us, we could embrace policies that verge on the punitive, coercive, illiberal. To avoid this we should appeal to the hopes of those we serve rather than to their fears, and work toward a public health that values joy and all the positive benefits that health can bring. In emphasizing this focus we can shape a public health that is more able to appeal to our better angels, moving toward creating a healthier world supported by liberal ideals.

It isn't always easy for us to lean into positivity. Our messaging seeks to curb behaviors that can lead to sickness and preventable harm, so it tends to involve statements that begin (implicitly), with "Thou shalt not." Thou shalt not drink. Thou shalt not smoke. Thou shalt not eat to excess. We mean these statements as a blueprint for behavior that supports a long, healthy life. Yet it is possible to read them as prohibitions against fun, against the pleasure and joy that are core to living that very life.

Some might dismiss this as merely a matter of tone, secondary to more urgent priorities. Yet the wrong tone risks alienating the very public we

are meant to serve, and in doing so it weakens the effectiveness of public health. Consider what we saw during COVID-19. The threat posed by
the pandemic meant that the population was receptive to the message of
public health, arguably as never before. Yet even in these circumstances
there was resistance. Such resistance—even in the midst of a pandemic—
suggests that some see public health primarily as an attempt to curtail
freedom and enjoyment and therefore to be resisted. The great irony of
this is that curtailing freedom and enjoyment is the precise opposite of
what public health should aspire to do. Our actual intent is to ensure that
as many people as possible are free to live long lives full of the activities and
interactions that bring happiness and meaning. Such lives are possible only
in the presence of health, of being free from the disease and preventable
harm that can stand between us and a happy life. And this outcome is possible only when it is supported by a liberal public health, one that eschews
coercion in favor of persuasion, the negative in favor of the positive.

Is there a better approach we can take? Can we invert our image so
that it better aligns with our mission to maximize happiness and help us
all fulfill our human potential? I suggest we can, by embracing three ideas.

First, we can advance a definition of health that is fundamentally positive. This means communicating that public health advice is meant to
enable enjoyment, not curtail it. As an illustration, let's compare public
health advice to the advice given by pool safety signs. I am always struck by
the way such signs tend to list prohibitions: "Do not drink the pool water,"
"Do not swim alone," "No diving in the shallow end." Such prohibitions are
all necessary and reasonable, yet their stern pronouncements are easy to
ignore, as many people do. Might it make a difference to include a friendly
request that captures the essence of why pool and people are there in the
first place? "Have fun in the water!" To put that on a sign even without
removing any of its other important warnings could do much to ensure
that the sign is noticed and the warnings heeded, to the ultimate good of all
the swimmers. It would also be something nice for them to see, a positive
note that keeps them safer. We could advance a public health that is much
like that sign, keeping core messaging intact while including positive elements that speak to the central reason we wish to be healthy: to live good
lives.

This leads to a second idea: We should promote health not as an end
in itself, but as a means to living a happy life. When we talk about health
solely as the prevention of disease, it is indeed disease that characterizes

much of our conversation. But when we regard health not as an end, but as a necessary step on the journey toward a full life, the conversation about health emphasizes all the positive factors that animate such a life. Talking about health in this way would represent a significant departure from the way most people discuss it. Our overwhelming investment in doctors and medicines in the United States reflects the high premium we put on health as an end in itself, for which no price is too high. Changing course will mean a fundamental shift in what we talk about when we talk about health. Key to creating this change will be using narrative and storytelling to broaden our imagination about what health is for. I favor the metaphor of investing in a car. Imagine buying a nice car and pouring money into its upkeep, ensuring that it will run smoothly, but then never taking it out of the garage. This car is like our health as we currently understand it. We take pains to keep the car in good shape but forget that the whole purpose of having a car is to travel. Public health, then, aims to keep the car in good shape while also building good roads, creating attractive scenery, and doing everything possible to ensure a pleasant journey. This is the kind of positive, aspirational story we should be telling to better engage with the public.

Finally, we can revisit the language of public health measures to emphasize the positive importance of health as a means of living a long, happy life. For example, we could revisit the concept of disability-adjusted life years (DALYs). DALYs is a common term in public health, defined as the combination of years of life lost owing to some disease or injury and years spent living with disability or suboptimal health as a consequence of such conditions. DALYs constitute a powerful tool for calculating the effects of various health problems. Yet they also further embed within the way we talk about health a focus on the disease we aim to prevent at the expense of the joy and pleasure we hope to enable. A helpful counterpoint would be measuring a combination of years of potential life gained and years spent in full health as a result of public health interventions. This could shift our focus from an exclusive concern with death and disease to one that also engages with the positive aspects of life that we hope to support through our work.

I will conclude with a literary reference that I think reflects these points well. The poet Hart Crane once wrote in a letter, "The poetry of negation is beautiful—alas, too dangerously so for one of my mind. But I am trying to break away from it. Perhaps this is useless, perhaps it is silly—but one *does* have joys. The vocabulary of damnations and prostrations has been developed at the expense of these other moods, however, so that it is hard to dance in proper measure."

I believe that the work of public health, in its emphasis on preventing disease rather than on enabling pleasure and joy, risks being seen as something like "the poetry of negation"—negation of the activities that bring pleasure and fun. In preventing disease, we should not lose sight of the fact that "one does have joys," and celebrating joy should be at the heart of the work of public health. Such a positive focus is essential to engaging more effectively with the populations we serve and supporting a liberal approach to our work. By balancing our emphasis on preventing sickness with an emphasis on enabling joy, we can become better at doing both, so that we can "dance in proper measure" toward the aim of supporting health.

SOURCES

"Disability-Adjusted Life Years (DALYs)." World Health Organization. https://www.who .int/data/gho/indicator-metadata-registry/imr-details/158. Accessed April 28, 2022.

Galea, S. Well: What We Need to Talk About When We Talk About Health. Oxford: Oxford University Press, 2019.

Georgia Pool Sign: Pool Risks (S2-2216). MyPoolSigns. https://www.mypoolsigns.com /georgia-pool-risks-sign/sku-s2-2216. Accessed April 28, 2022.

Hagell, A., and R. Cheung. "Using DALYs to Understand Young People's Health." Nuffield Trust. https://www.nuffieldtrust.org.uk/resource/using-dalys-to-understand-young -people-s-health. Published February 21, 2019. Accessed April 28, 2022.

Hammer, L. Hart Crane and Allen Tate: Janus-Faced Modernism. Princeton, NJ: Princeton University Press, 2017.

A PLAYBOOK FOR
BALANCING THE MORAL AND
EMPIRICAL CASES FOR HEALTH

At core, public health aspires to strike a balance between the moral and the empirical cases for maintaining good health. I have long thought that at times public health has not gone far enough in advancing the moral case. This belief has motivated me to argue in the past for an epidemiology of consequence. In that instance, and in subsequent writing with Katherine Keyes, I have argued for an approach to public health that—guided by the moral imperative of generating good health for the greatest number of people—aims to apply its empirical knowledge to the pursuit of a healthier world. This means giving priority, on moral and empirical grounds, to engaging with the issues that matter most for health, through research guided above all by the demands of human need, with an eye toward doing the most practical good.

In recent years the pendulum has indeed swung this way, toward a public health emphasizing consequences and guided by the moral case for health. During COVID-19 our collective balance, our effort to find the right mix of moral and empirical motivation, was tested as perhaps never before. This is understandable. Consequences for health are by definition matters of life and death that concern the well-being of everyone—both present and future generations—and that matter with particular urgency when we are all vulnerable, and some of us especially so. COVID was particularly troubling because we often found ourselves needing to make a moral case before we could gather empirical evidence. If our arguments are to successfully support health, I continue to find it important to make sure they aspire to strike a balance between the moral and the empirical, reflecting the pragmatic realities and trade-offs inherent in doing so. This is particularly true when our pursuit of moral clarity tips us into an illiberal engagement with issues. Such thinking can cause us to minimize inconvenient facts or to demonize intellectual opponents. This risk makes it all the more important that we find ways to balance the moral and empirical

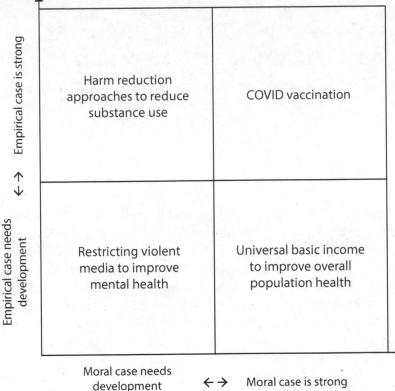

cases for health, toward ensuring that our approach is informed by the proper measure of each.

The grid shown here is meant to help us visualize how we might approach this. It was inspired by Donald Stokes's book *Pasteur's Quadrant: Basic Science and Technological Innovation*. Each of the grid's quadrants contains an action that could arguably help create a healthier world. The quadrant at the top left shows steps for which the empirical case is strong but the moral case needs development. The bottom left shows steps for which both the empirical and moral cases need development. The bottom right shows steps for which the moral case is strong but the empirical case needs development. The top right shows steps for which both the empirical and moral cases are strong—this is where all our arguments should aspire to live.

As an example, I have placed in the top left quadrant harm-reduction approaches to reducing substance use, where the empirical case is strong but the moral case needs development. There is some evidence that these approaches to substance use, such as needle exchanges, can indeed reduce harm. Despite these data, the moral case for these approaches is complicated by the impression that they seem to condone substance use by aiming to mitigate harm rather than by taking a zero-tolerance approach. This places them in a category where they are supported by data but not yet by a fully articulated moral case that has cleared the way for their widespread use.

Below harm reduction is the case for restricting violent media to improve mental health. This reflects a situation where both the empirical and moral arguments need development. At a surface level, the idea of restricting violent media can seem to have merit. We know, for example, that images of trauma can contribute the development of depression and PTSD. Yet from an empirical perspective there are not enough data to conclude that banning such media would be an unalloyed good for mental health. Some data suggest, for example, that video games—a frequently cited form of media that is at times violent—can benefit well-being. At the same time, the moral case for banning such media is complicated because such a ban resembles censorship. Given the difficult ethical questions surrounding such a step, a potential restriction on violent media occupies the weakest position on the grid, with little moral or empirical support.

In the bottom right quadrant is the case for embracing universal basic income (UBI). Here the moral argument is strong but the empirical case needs development. UBI offers much potential to help create a healthier country. I have often written that health depends on access to the material resources money buys. But many lack access to these resources because socioeconomic structures favor people who already have much and disfavor those who have less. Thus it is easy to make the moral case for UBI. Yet while we do know much about the link between money and health, we know little about the link between UBI specifically and health. Because UBI hasn't yet been enacted on a national scale in the United States, we don't have data on how it would affect health in the near and long term. We can hypothesize, with fair confidence, that it would significantly improve health, but until we have data we cannot truly know. This means that although the moral case for UBI is strong, we should proceed with due humility about the limits of our current understanding of its enactment on a national scale.

Finally, in the top right quadrant there is the case for COVID vaccination. Of all the arguments presented on the grid, this one is best positioned, with the moral and empirical cases equally strong. The data on vaccine effectiveness are clear, as are the data on the danger of going unvaccinated. Equally clear is the moral importance of getting vaccinated both for our own sakes and for the sake of our community. While the strength of the case for vaccination was, sadly, not enough to persuade everyone to get the shot, this hesitancy is not for lack of overwhelming support of vaccination by both the data and the urgings of basic morality.

Note that, even as we strive to balance the moral and empirical cases for health, we need not wait until this balance has been achieved before making our arguments. Often the empirical components of an argument exist long before a sense of moral urgency reaches a point where it can be fused, in the public debate, with the data that support it. When the United States renewed the conversation about race in the summer of 2020, for example, the topic was informed by years of data reflecting the link between racism and poor health. We in public health possessed these data, but they had not yet gained the collective moral urgency needed to truly inform the national conversation—until all of a sudden they did.

Germane to this, economist Milton Friedman once said, "Only a crisis—actual or perceived—produces real change. When that crisis occurs, the actions that are taken depend on the ideas that are lying around. That, I believe, is our basic function: to develop alternatives to existing policies, to keep them alive and available until the politically impossible becomes the politically inevitable."

I realize it is somewhat ironic to quote Friedman in an essay that aims to help advance progressive reforms the libertarian economist might not have approved of. Yet I think his words are relevant. They speak to the core importance of laying well in advance the empirical groundwork for the policies that support health. We can then elevate these data in the public debate, with an eye toward sparking the moral urgency to match the force of our data. Notably, this is possible only in the presence of a liberal public health dedicated, above all else, to the reasoned pursuit of health. Both the moral and the empirical cases are ultimately necessary if we are to make the strongest possible argument for a healthier world. Aspiring to strike this balance should be at the heart of our thinking about how we create such a world.

SOURCES

Friedman, M. Quotation by Milton Freidman. Goodreads. https://www.goodreads.com /quotes/110844-only-a-crisis---actual-or-perceived---produces-real-change. Accessed April 28, 2022.

Galea, S. "An Argument for a Consequentialist Epidemiology." *American Journal of Epidemiology* 178, no. 8 (2013): 1185–91.

———. "On Economic Justice." Boston University School of Public Health. https://www.bu.edu/sph/news/articles/2017/on-economic-justice/. Published January 29, 2017. Accessed April 28, 2022.

———. "The Stimulus Is Necessary Medicine." *Healthiest Goldfish* (blog), February 6, 2021. https://sandrogalea.substack.com/p/the-stimulus-is-necessary-medicine. Accessed April 28, 2022.

———. *Well: What We Need to Talk About When We Talk About Health.* Oxford: Oxford University Press, 2019

Johannes, N., M. Vuorre, and A. K. Przybylski. "Video Game Play Is Positively Correlated with Well-Being." *Royal Society Open Science* 8, no. 2, (2021): 1–14.

Keyes, K., and S. Galea. "What Matters Most: Quantifying an Epidemiology of Consequence." *Annals of Epidemiology* 25, no. 5 (2021): 305–11.

Marlatt, G. A., and K. Witkiewitz. "Harm Reduction Approaches to Alcohol Use: Health Promotion, Prevention, and Treatment." *Addictive Behaviors* 27, no. 6 (2002): 867–86.

Ritter, A., and J. A. Cameron. "A Review of the Efficacy and Effectiveness of Harm Reduction Strategies for Alcohol, Tobacco and Illicit Drugs." *Drug and Alcohol Review* 25, no. 6 (2006): 611–24.

Stokes, D. E. *Pasteur's Quadrant: Basic Science and Technological Innovation.* Washington, DC: Brookings Institution Press, 1997.

THE FALSE CHOICE OF DIVERSITY AND INCLUSION VERSUS THE PURSUIT OF EXCELLENCE

In April 2021 United Airlines pledged to train five thousand new pilots by 2030, no fewer than half of them women or people of color. With this announcement came pushback, including a common objection to efforts at diversity and inclusion that extends back to the start of debate concerning initiatives like affirmative action: that, in making room for historically underrepresented groups, we risk elevating concerns about identity above a commitment to excellence, even though the intention is to bring in the best people regardless of skin color, sex or gender identity, or other characteristics that have led to past marginalization. These concerns were particularly potent with regard to the airline industry, where anything less than excellence in the cockpit could put lives at risk.

United's pledge aligned with other welcome efforts to promote greater diversity and inclusion within organizations. This movement has been a long time coming and is something I have cared about throughout my career. Yet as the elevation of diversity and inclusion has become part of the fabric of more and more institutions, we more frequently hear the objection that diversity and inclusion conflict with excellence, undermining the meritocracy that sustains effective organizations. This objection has implications for health. Building a healthier world depends on pursuing excellence within a range of organizations, from academia to government to the infrastructure of public health. As this necessity intersects with the growing embrace of diversity and inclusion within these bodies, it is important not to shy away from engaging with objections to this focus. It is worth asking if these efforts, laudable in theory, may in practice lead to illiberal approaches. For our institutions to be strong enough to support health, those working within them must be able to engage with this question. With that in mind, I will share a few thoughts about the supposed conflict between excellence and diversity, and about what it means for liberalism within public health.

It's first worth asking, What are the practical effects of diversity within organizations? According to a 2017 analysis by McKinsey and Company, companies in the top quartile for gender diversity on their executive teams were 21 percent likelier to enjoy financial performance above the national industry median. Companies in the top quartile for ethnic diversity on their executive teams were 33 percent likelier to do so.

These data support what many of us consider intuitive about greater diversity in organizations: it is a positive influence. Diversity means more potential for new ideas and approaches—the lifeblood of any dynamic group. It can also reduce the groupthink that can result in missteps. If everyone thinks the same way, no one is in a position to raise the alarm when the group is moving in the wrong direction. Diversity can help ensure that groups will include perspectives outside the majority, which can keep an organization from falling prey to the blind spots that can lead to poor decisions. This is also a core function of liberalism, which works to accommodate many perspectives, allowing for broad disagreement within an atmosphere of mutual toleration and respect. Ideally, diversity permeates and strengthens such a context, helping to support a liberal public health.

A brief story will illustrate the importance of diversity. Imagine there are two ships. On one ship the crew lacks diversity, with all the sailors sharing a similar background and philosophy about the sea. On the other ship there is true diversity, with sailors from different backgrounds and different perspectives. On the first ship the crew and captain are unanimous about the direction they are heading, with everyone agreeing it is the right course. Unfortunately, they are wrong. They sail into a storm and sink. The other ship also briefly heads toward the storm, but because of its diversity, a number of sailors onboard question their initial course. After a brief debate in which everyone is included, the captain in consultation with the crew decides to change course, avoiding the storm and eventually arriving safely at their destination. Diversity has saved their voyage.

Note how this story helps define both diversity and inclusion, two words that are often used together. Diversity is the presence in a given space of people of different backgrounds, perspectives, and identities. Inclusion is their full participation in whatever is happening in that space. For example, the second ship was diverse because the crew had many sailors of different backgrounds. It was inclusive because they all were engaged in the conversation about where the ship should go. Diversity is always a worthwhile goal, but unless it is a prelude to inclusion, it cannot fully support spaces where people of different backgrounds can come together and flourish. In a sense, a balance of diversity and inclusion mirrors the functioning of a liberal society. Without inclusion, diversity cannot truly flourish: it may look nice, but it will remain superficial unless all are included. Likewise, if we abandon liberalism in public health, we may continue to resemble our former selves, but it will be a surface resemblance, without the core values that once enabled our efforts.

The story of the ships, and the data supporting diversity's salutary effect on organizations, reflects the way—far from undermining excellence—diversity and inclusion are core to supporting it. Expanding on this, three points help support, I think, a vision of diversity and inclusion that is central to advancing the excellence necessary for building a healthier world.

First, much depends on how we define excellence. Certainly there are some cases where excellence must be narrowly defined. For the pilot, for example, excellence means being able to consistently provide a safe flight for passengers and crew, and there's no getting around this definition. But in other areas there is ample room to rethink our definition of excellence. Consider rocket science. In many respects excellence is quite specific in how it supports this field. The equations that send a rocket into space are not subject to different interpretations, and there is no margin of error in their use. However, there is much room for diversity of thought about the type of rockets used and their potential destinations. Returning to the ship example, the key contribution of diversity was not in rethinking how boats work, but in envisioning a better course for the voyage. When excellence is defined in these terms—still as a meritocratic pursuit, but as one less bound by settled habits and conventional wisdom—it can help our endeavors reach new heights.

Second, just as we can be well served by reimagining our notions of excellence, we can also benefit from rethinking just what we mean by diversity. We often find ourselves stuck with a narrow conception. In some ways this habit of thought reflects something very positive. Acknowledging that for generations paths to success were closed to people from certain identity groups, and that we are now trying to correct this injustice, is very much to the good. But confusion can arise when we give the impression that diversity is entirely a matter of making sure to represent a certain composition of identity groups, excluding all other considerations. Besides the fact that such a reductionist approach fails to account for inclusion, we might ask, Is this true diversity? Of course as a baseline introduction it is a kind of diversity, certainly better than what we've had the past. But it is also possible to think more expansively about diversity. The crew of the second ship saved themselves not just because of their different backgrounds, but because everybody's perspective was heard.

This diversity of thought allowed them to recognize when the group was in danger of making an error and to change course. A key benefit of bringing together people with different experiences and identities is viewpoint diversity—the different perspectives their unique experiences can contribute. This diversity includes different opinions, skill sets, political beliefs, and spiritual outlooks. Creating space for viewpoint diversity is in many ways the most difficult element of supporting diversity, because we must make room for those we may disagree with. Yet if we shy away from creating this space, we leave undone the full work of diversity and inclusion. We also risk perpetuating feedback loops and the groupthink that can characterize increasingly politicized public health institutions. For this reason, diversity and inclusion are well served by operating within a liberal framework where everyone has a fundamental right to speak and to be heard. At times it can seem that diversity demands quieting certain voices, such as those that do not regard diversity as an unalloyed good. Yet through the lens of liberalism we can see that true diversity depends on including such voices, with the understanding that in an open marketplace of ideas controversial views can coexist with ideas we may find more palatable.

This leads to the third point, a caution against the zero-sum thinking that can characterize our view of the relation between diversity and excellence. Just as viewpoint diversity means rejecting the zero-sum thinking that does not tolerate competing ideas, the broader pursuit of diversity means accepting that diversity and excellence are not in any way mutually exclusive. Indeed, the idea of inclusive excellence has made steady inroads in the conversation about diversity, particularly in academia. Given the data in support of diversity's positive effects on organizations and teams, it is clear that embracing diversity need not involve trade-offs at the expense of excellence. Core to this is ensuring that the diversity we embrace is full diversity, including diversity of viewpoints. When diversity is able to flourish, when it can support a full range of identities, backgrounds, perspectives, and intellectual leanings, it is poised to be a powerful force for maximizing human potential in any setting.

Why does this matter? Why is it so important that we make a robust case for diversity and inclusion by engaging with objections to it? It matters because diversity and inclusion are central to creating a healthier world. Fundamentally, health is concerned with supporting the well-being of populations; and by "populations," I mean as many people as possible. We cannot effectively promote health among such a diverse constituency without reflecting, and learning from, the people we serve. Diversity and inclusion are also core to a liberal public health, helping us achieve excellence by listening to a range of perspectives, stress-testing ideas through a robust public debate in which everybody can have a say.

SOURCES

American Association of Colleges and Universities. https://www.aacu.org. Accessed April 28, 2022.

Hunt, V., L. Yee, S. Prince, and S. Dixon-Fyle. "Delivering through Diversity." McKinsey and Company. https://www.mckinsey.com/business-functions/people-and-organizational-performance/our-insights/delivering-through-diversity. Published January 18, 2018. Accessed April 28, 2022.

"Inclusive Excellence 1 and 2." Howard Hughes Medical Institute. https://www.hhmi.org/science-education/programs/inclusive-excellence-1-2. Accessed April 28, 2022.

Rock, D., and H. Grant. "Why Diverse Teams Are Smarter." *Harvard Business Review*, November 4, 2016. https://hbr.org/2016/11/why-diverse-teams-are-smarter. Accessed April 28, 2022.

Singh, S. "United Airlines Hits Back at Pilot Training Diversity Criticism." *Simple Flying*, April 7, 2021. https://simpleflying.com/united-airlines-pilot-diversity-critisism/. Accessed April 28, 2022.

OUR PLACE IN THE
NATURAL ORDER OF THINGS

I have long believed there is a fundamental insecurity at the heart of illiberalism, perhaps most apparent in the stifling of free speech and debate. When we rush to muzzle dissent, our actions can betray a subconscious doubt about our own position. If we are secure in the reasoned basis for what we believe, why should we fear debate? Likewise, why should a self-confident public health, secure in its place in the natural order, turn toward illiberalism? That we have at times done so suggests we are perhaps not as secure as we might think. Because we have forgotten our roots, our deepest values, we turn to politics and ideology to orient ourselves in a complex, changing world. This turn—understandably human as it is—can perpetuate illiberalism within our field. This is not true only of public health, of course. History has shown that when societies are insecure, they are liable to be less healthy and more susceptible to illiberalism. It is better for everyone, then, if we can each live secure in our place in the natural order, supported by the socioeconomic assets that make this so.

What, then, are the values and aspirations we should foreground as we try to create such a world, where we all can be secure?

One way to consider this question is by thinking about parallel universes, which in my disciplinary home—epidemiology—we call counterfactuals. These counterfactuals allow us to model the way introducing a given variable might shape health. We do so by comparing a real world where someone might, say, smoke with a counterfactual universe where that same person, *with everything else held exactly the same*, does not smoke. This allows us to compare counterfactual universes where everything is the same except that one variable. We can then conclude that if the person we are observing gets lung cancer in the universe where she smokes—and avoids it in the universe where she does not—we might say with some confidence that smoking causes lung cancer.

Of course this model has limitations. For one thing, it's fictional—it doesn't exist. For another, it's hard to conceptualize a universe where everything is the same save one detail. And this paradigm seems even less grounded in reality when we are framing more complex variables such as race or gender. But notwithstanding all this, counterfactuals remain an invaluable tool for conceptualizing the conditions that shape health. For example, it is easy to imagine future historians using counterfactuals to parse what we did wrong, and right, during COVID-19.

So now let's run a counterfactual experiment. Imagine two identical people living in universes that are the same save for one key detail, a detail that is core to the ability to live a healthy life: in one universe the person is secure in her place in the natural order of things, whereas in the other she is not. By secure I mean possessing enough socioeconomic advantages to know, in her heart of hearts, that no matter how bad life gets, ultimately she will probably be OK. This security means the difference, for example, between sudden illness being a hardship and its being a calamity, or between losing a few thousand dollars being a temporary setback and its extinguishing her quality of life.

This security can come from many places. Perhaps it comes from wealth, which can buffer us against catastrophe. Perhaps it comes from family connections, or skin color. Feeling supported by the natural order, rather than at odds with it, is a complex, often intangible good. It seems to me that it is almost invariably reflected in the long-term trajectory of one's life. It changes everything. Knowing that one has an assured place in the natural order makes one more willing to take risks, to venture ideas, to travel, to speak truth to power, to take actions that require deeply internalized convictions. Ultimately such actions amount to a fully realized life and the sense of well-being such a life supports, a sense that is necessary for health. We can imagine, then, how much healthier the subject of our experiment likely is in the universe where she feels secure in the natural order of things.

It strikes me, then, that if we want to create a healthy world, it must be a world where feeling secure is not a privilege enjoyed by the few, but a right claimed by everyone. And that this matters in this way, and does so tremendously, places it at the heart of achieving our aspirations of public health.

This conclusion echoes a famous thought experiment developed by the philosopher John Rawls, in which we are asked to design a new society. The society can take the form of monarchy, dictatorship, democracy—any form of political or economic organization we want. It can be equal or unequal, just or exploitative. The key point is that, although we are free to design this society, we are not allowed to know in advance what our own place in the order of things will be. We could be in a position of privilege or we could be at the bottom of the socioeconomic ladder. Rawls called this position of incomplete knowledge the Veil of Ignorance. Because we are designing our society from behind this veil, it behooves us to build a world that is as equitable as possible, where all are secure in their places in the natural order.

How might we go about doing this in the world we have? How can we move toward this aspiration? Broadly speaking, I believe we need to take three steps.

First, we need to ensure that all people have access to the resources that can allow them to feel secure—physically and financially—in the natural order of things. There are a number of ways to go about this, but ambitious federal investment strikes me as the necessary condition for them all. We can have conversations about the trajectory of spending—what proportion should go directly to individuals and what should be used to support community investment, the social safety net, and other public goods—but no matter where the money goes, it should mark a paradigm shift in federal investment toward a bolder vision for providing Americans with material aid.

Second, we need to create a foundation of compassion, to support a world that protects rather than castigates its citizens. In talking about compassion, I mean compassion in the sense that Martin Luther King Jr. described when he said, "True compassion is more than flinging a coin to a beggar; it comes to see that an edifice which produces beggars needs restructuring." Creating a world that lets everyone feel secure takes structural changes. Compassion helps us see where these changes are necessary and motivates us to make them.

Finally, we need to stop marginalizing people based on their identity. This means creating a world where we all can thrive as individuals, regardless of sex/gender, skin color, or socioeconomic status. At a time when identity looms so large, transcending these categories may be the most difficult of the steps I have suggested. In a sense, the categories of identity have become a new Veil of Ignorance, with outward appearances preventing us from seeing other people's true individuality and preventing our own individuality from being seen. It is perhaps tempting to maintain categories of identity as a means of navigating the world, even as a means of improving it, yet this risks obscuring the individuality of those we encounter. Just as we must live in the world we create from behind the classic

Veil of Ignorance, not knowing in advance what part of society we will occupy, we must now live in a world veiled by the prominence of identity, and we cannot know in advance who we might otherwise have met on their own terms, by looking beyond reductive categories. If we shape a society around identity, we risk fraying the ties between individuals, ties that are essential to supporting our sense of belonging, our sense of solid ground in a changing, challenging world. This is especially true in light of the divisions of recent years, when grievances based mainly on identity have done much to drive us apart.

This argues for a liberal public health agenda, centrally characterized by inclusivity and compassion, that aims to help everyone feel secure in the natural order. Public health is organized around the aspiration of universal health, which we cannot achieve as long as we have parallel universes where some people feel on sure footing in our society while others do not. Ensuring that everyone feels secure means providing a foundation of material support we can all stand on. And as we build this foundation, we should support the groups that have been made disproportionately vulnerable to poor health by historical and socioeconomic forces, while taking care that this necessary focus does not prevent us from seeing groups as a collection of individuals with their own unique perspectives and experiences. Fundamentally, being secure in our world must lie at the heart of our aspirations for health; it is up to us to advocate for the conditions that make this so for all.

SOURCES

BBC Radio 4. "The Veil of Ignorance" (video). YouTube. https://www.youtube.com/watch?v=A8GDEaJtbq4. Published April 8, 2015. Accessed April 29, 2022.

King, M. L. Quotation by Martin Luther King Jr. Goodreads. https://www.goodreads.com/quotes/19814-true-compassion-is-more-than-flinging-a-coin-to-a. Accessed April 29, 2022.

Stein, V., and D. Dobrijevic. "Do Parallel Universes Exist? We Might Live in a Multiverse." Space.com. https://www.space.com/32728-parallel-universes.html. Published November 3, 2021. Accessed April 29, 2022.

WHAT DO WE WANT FROM
OUR POLITICAL SYSTEM?

Addressing the challenge of illiberalism in public health is in some ways about more than just our field. The illiberalism we have seen in public health is arguably a symptom of a broader illiberalism that some find an attractive alternative to our current political culture. Calling out illiberalism in public health, then, is part of a broader conversation about what we want from our political system. Do we want our politics to be liberal or illiberal? If we want a liberal politics, it's worth asking how we can optimize our current political system toward supporting health for the greatest number of people, to minimize the discontent that can make illiberalism appealing. With this in mind, here are some thoughts on how we can shape such a system so that our liberal model remains viable and robust, supportive of a healthier world.

It is one of the most-used aphorisms in public health: "Politics [is] nothing but medicine at a larger scale." That phrase comes from Rudolf Virchow, one of the founders of modern pathology, who also played a key role in the development of social medicine. Virchow became convinced that the underlying reasons for health gaps were social and economic inequities, leading him to participate in the revolutions of 1848, among other progressive efforts of his time. In articulating a central role for politics in the health conversation, Virchow was in many respects decades ahead of his time, and his work led directly to much of the modern discussion about the role politics plays in shaping health.

Politics, perhaps most easily defined as the art and science of governance that allows us to live together, unquestionably shapes health. And in my assessment we in public health have been—correctly—increasingly vocal about this role. Perhaps in direct reaction to the Trump administration, which was responsible for a set of policies that in the main were detrimental to health, we have had a growing chorus of voices arguing for the importance of thinking about politics when we think about health. And given the more visible role of public health in the public arena owing to a world-stopping pandemic, it is possible that these voices now have more weight. But as we increasingly engage in urging politics to consider health as part of its core mission, we could also benefit from clarity about what we are trying to achieve through politics. It is easy to argue against, say, neoliberal ideas, which we reflexively sense will cause us to underinvest in health—even if, I suggest, the evidence here is not at all clear. But it is harder to think about what we are trying to achieve through our political system. Perhaps being clearer on that may help us focus our advocacy efforts, as well as the scholarship that can guide how we engage with politics to begin with. Such clarity may also lend more sophistication to our engagement with politics, so that rather than finding ourselves a mere extension of a political party, we maintain our independence of thought and the freedom to pursue data wherever they lead.

I have come to think there are three areas that should guide what we want out of a politics that creates a better, healthier world.

We want our politics to create the *assets* that can generate health for as many people as possible and can narrow health gaps. This may be the clearest aspiration we can have for politics, and it will be familiar to many. We know that health is generated by the conditions of where we work, live, and play. That leads naturally to the understanding that health is a function of our access to these conditions, and of whether they are health generating or health harming. Of course, I am using the word assets very broadly. Assets themselves help: that is to say, having the money to buy things that make us healthy. Even more broadly, health-generating assets include quality neighborhoods, gender equity, a clean environment, and so on, helped by livable wages and wealth. The link between having assets and having health is captured in a long list of writings on health, anchored by fundamental-cause thinking that suggests simply that access to these assets is foundational to health. It is therefore this exact disinvestment in these assets that made the Trump administration so harmful to health. When we stop investing in the conditions that create a better world by broadening access to the assets that generate health, we also stop building health. This is also why the United States has fallen behind peer countries on health, with our life expectancy now being up to five years lower than that of the best-performing nations, despite our spending more on health than anyone else. At a simple level, our politics has not been investing in the assets that create health, and so our health has suffered. An important corollary is that inequitable distribution of assets leads directly to health inequities. The poorest 80 percent of Americans are falling even further behind the richest 20 percent. Black Americans continue to have life expectancy about four years lower than that of white Americans, and in a time of pandemic they have had twice the mortality rate from COVID-19. These differences are driven largely by inequitable access to assets. Therefore assets are instrumental to health, and both those assets and our access to them are determined in large part by our politics. We want, then, a political system that invests in the assets that generate health, and that does so in an equitable way, as a means of narrowing health gaps.

We also want our politics to create *opportunities* for us, as citizens, to live fully realized lives. Whether those of us interested in health see this as an important part of our mission depends in no small part on how we see the role of health. If we were interested only in health in itself, we might be willing to constrain opportunities for living just to achieve health. To my mind, however, health is a means, not an end. That suggests that we should work to ensure healthier populations so that all can choose to live their lives with purpose and meaning. We know, in turn, that living with purpose is associated with lower mortality. This means that creating such opportunities should be central to any political system that cares about health. Yes, there are times when in order to generate health we are willing to constrain some opportunities for expression—it seems well worthwhile, for example, to enforce wearing seatbelts to reduce motor vehicle fatalities. But, fundamentally, health should be in service of opportunity, and we should aim for political systems that act accordingly. This is consistent with a liberal vision for both politics and public health. In both cases we are well served by being judicious about the constraints we must sometimes advocate for, while emphasizing the broader benefits of the freedom and opportunities that come with living a healthy life.

Last, but certainly not least, we want our politics to allow us all to live with *dignity*. I realize we don't talk about this much in the context of health, but it has always seemed to me that the goal of concepts such as human rights is indeed to ensure that we can all live with dignity. Understanding dignity as a belief that we all have intrinsic value linked to our humanity suggests that we should be working toward systems that promote such value, independent of any identity—be it race, country of birth, income, class—other than our shared humanity. This has enormous implications concerning our priorities for our political systems. It means elevating systems that promote respect for all, predicated on what we have in common, not on our differences. We have already seen in the past few years the perils of excluding so many in our population from the opportunity to live lives of dignity and respect. It is not a stretch to note that this led to Donald Trump's election as president. It also pushes us to ensure that our efforts to promote a pluralist world that recognizes and values our differences do not come at the expense of efforts to elevate our shared humanity, efforts that encourage us to see health as a public good and not to have health left-behinds. It is also worth noting that the notion of dignity—the idea that individuals have certain basic rights—is core to the philosophical basis of our liberal system. Echoes of it can be heard in everything from the US Declaration of Independence to the Universal Declaration of Human Rights. When we turn away from liberalism, we risk undermining the dignity that an effective politics, and public health, should support.

Working to define our politics in this way is, to my thinking, how public health should be engaging with politics—as opposed to an engagement that sees us as mere partisan actors. Rather than constantly jockeying for partisan advantage, we should embrace a deeper engagement with politics, one that helps redefine what our political system can do, orienting it toward health.

Taken together, an aspiration that allows the generation of assets, opportunity, and dignity for all has implications for the types of political systems we encourage, aiming to generate a healthier world. For example, I would not consider a system of central political and economic control as particularly commensurate with creating opportunity, and clearly a basic shortcoming of a completely market-driven economy is that it not infrequently robs people of dignity. But our actions in promoting health also risk forgetting why we are doing what we are doing when we turn toward illiberalism.

SOURCES

Abdalla, S. M., N. Maani, C. K. Ettman, and S. Galea. "Claiming Health as a Public Good in the Post-COVID-19 Era." *Development* (Rome) 63, nos. 2–4 (2020): 200–204.

Abdalla, S. M., S. Yu, and S. Galea. "Trends in Cardiovascular Disease Prevalence by Income Level in the United States." *JAMA Network Open* 3, no. 9 (2020): e2018150.

Alimujiang, A., A. Wiensch, J. Boss, N. L. Fleischer, A. M. Mondul, K. McKlean, et al. "Association between Life Purpose and Mortality among US Adults Older Than 50 Years." *JAMA Network Open* 2, no. 5 (2019): e194270.

"American Health Care: Health Spending and the Federal Budget." Committee for a Responsible Federal Budget. https://www.crfb.org/papers/american-health-care-health-spending-and-federal-budget. Published May 16, 2018. Accessed April 29, 2022.

Galea, S. "Gender Equity and the Health of Populations." Boston University School of Public Health. https://www.bu.edu/sph/news/articles/2016/gender-equity-and-the-health-of-populations/. Published March 6, 2016. Accessed April 29, 2022.

————. "How the Trump Administration's Policies May Harm the Public's Health." *Milbank Quarterly* 95, no. 2 (2017): 229–32.

————. "Learning from November 3: A Wake-Up Call for Public Health." *Milbank Quarterly*, November 4, 2020. https://www.milbank.org/quarterly/opinions/learning-from -november-3-a-wake-up-call-for-public-health/. Accessed April 29, 2022.

————. "On Economic Justice." Boston University School of Public Health. https://www .bu.edu/sph/news/articles/2017/on-economic-justice/. Published January 29, 2017. Accessed April 29, 2022.

————. *Well: What We Need to Talk About When We Talk About Health*. Oxford: Oxford University Press, 2019.

Galea, S., C. K. Ettman, and D. Vlahov. *Urban Health*. Oxford: Oxford University Press, 2019.

Galea, S., and J. Levy. "There Is No Public Health without Environmental Health." Boston University School of Public Health. https://www.bu.edu/sph/news/articles/2018 /there-is-no-public-health-without-environmental-health/. Published October 26, 2018. Accessed April 29, 2022.

Galea, S., and R. D. Vaughan. "Galea and Vaughan Respond." *American Journal of Public Health* 109, no. 12 (2019): e1–e2.

Himmelstein, D. U., S. Woolhandler, R. Cooney, M. McKee, and R. Horton. "The *Lancet* Commission on Public Policy and Health in the Trump Era." *Lancet* 392, no. 10152 (2018): 993–95.

Hunter, E. L. "Politics and Public Health—Engaging the Third Rail." *Journal of Public Health Management and Practice* 22, no. 5 (2016): 436–41.

Link, B. G., and J. Phelan. "Social Conditions as Fundamental Causes of Disease." *Journal of Health and Social Behavior*, 1995, special issue, 80–94.

Maani, N., and S. Galea. "COVID-19 and Underinvestment in the Health of the US Population." *Milbank Quarterly* 98, no. 2 (2020): 239–49.

Mackenbach, J. P. "Politics Is Nothing but Medicine at a Larger Scale: Reflections on Public Health's Biggest Idea." *Journal of Epidemiology and Community Health* 63, no. 3 (2009): 181–84.

Neuman, S. "COVID-19 Death Rate for Black Americans Twice That for Whites, New Report Says." *NPR*, August 13, 2020. https://www.npr.org/sections/coronavirus-live-up dates/2020/08/13/902261618/covid-19-death-rate-for-black-americans-twice-that-for -whites-new-report-says. Accessed April 29, 2022.

Ortaliza, J., G. Ramirez, V. Satheeskumar, and K. Amin. "How Does U.S. Life Expectancy Compare to Other Countries?" Health System Tracker. https://www.healthsystem tracker.org/chart-collection/u-s-life-expectancy-compare-countries/. Published September 28, 2021. Accessed April 29, 2022.

"Revolutions of 1848." Wikipedia. https://en.wikipedia.org/wiki/Revolutions_of_1848. Updated April 20, 2022. Accessed April 29, 2022.

Roberts, M., E. N. Reither, and S. Lim. "Contributors to the Black-White Life Expectancy Gap in Washington D.C." *Nature Scientific Reports* 10, no. 13416 (2020): 1–12.

Tracy, M., M. E. Kruk, C. Harper, and S. Galea. "Neo-liberal Economic Practices and Population Health: A Cross-National Analysis, 1980–2004." *Health Economics, Policy and Law* 5, no. 2 (2010): 171–99.

"What Is Human Dignity? Common Definitions." Human Rights Careers. https://www .humanrightscareers.com/issues/definitions-what-is-human-dignity/. Accessed April 29, 2022.

THE ROLE OF EXPERTS AND COMMUNITY VOICES BOTH

In recent years there has been much interest in elevating voices that have historically been marginalized in the public debate and in the academic spaces tasked with generating ideas. This reflects the growing, and welcome, understanding that for a long time such voices had been shut out of these conversations. Correcting this omission is not just an effort to address a historical wrong; it also reflects an acknowledgment that the lack of these voices may have set back our progress toward greater understanding of our science and our world. Efforts to align contemporary expertise with a more just approach to the production of knowledge aim in part to shape a fuller, richer science, drawing on the best of many traditions. Such efforts, then, are aspirational, prompted by our hopes for a better world and better science. And, broadly speaking, an expansive approach to alternative systems of understanding falls well within a liberal framework for inquiry. In the spirit of self-examination, however, it is worth asking if there are ways this approach, reexamining as it does core methodologies of the scientific process, could in any way misalign with them and the liberal inheritance they reflect. Asking this question can help us continue needed reappraisals of our reasoning in ways that respect the voices of both experts and the wider communities we serve.

First let's look at some of these reappraisals. One example is the growing interest in incorporating within academic disciplines indigenous "ways of knowing," with the aim of listening to alternative sources of knowledge and wisdom that may fall outside more established processes for generating new data. At the same time that we have seen a shift toward new ways of generating and classifying knowledge, we have seen questioning of more established models of expertise. On the right, this has come largely from a populist revolt against "elites" and their perceived tendency to claim their expertise—which some critics might call mere credentialism—as a mandate to govern from on high. On the left it has been characterized by a perspective that regards some of what we call knowledge as fundamentally compromised, emerging as it did from systems of inquiry developed and sustained by people whose privilege was at times supported by exploiting marginalized communities.

Just as science is reconsidering the use of indigenous knowledge and more subjective forms of experience in the pursuit of truth, within public health we have long sought to elevate the voices of the communities we serve—aiming to partner with them in creating a healthier world—even if we have frequently fallen short of that goal. It is not enough to simply design public health interventions and attempt to impose them from above, nor is it enough to assume that we, as a field, always know what is best for a given population. Rather, we need not just to listen to the populations we serve, but to actively ensure that they are represented within the ranks of public health itself, so that building a healthier world is truly a collaborative process in which we all work together to support the common good.

Yet the elevation of community voices has at times faced criticism. The core of this criticism is that, in making room for alternative approaches to the generation of knowledge in scientific and academic spaces, we risk undermining the core methodologies that support expertise—methodologies that emerged from the Enlightenment and the intellectual currents that animated what has become our liberal system. To the extent that such an approach reflects a politically progressive project, as it generally does, it can also underlie the broader perception that science has become politicized in ways that undermine its effectiveness as a knowledge-generating discipline. This prompts the question, Does making space for community voices necessarily mean dismissing more established forms of expertise? Or can we strike a balance between these means of understanding the world, with both animating our pursuit of health and coexisting within a liberal framework? To answer these questions, let's consider the arguments for each of these approaches to generating knowledge.

It is perhaps intuitive to begin with the importance of an understanding that is based on identity and the inherited knowledge of community. We all know the value of subjective experience, that certain truths are accessible only through personally walking a certain path in life. This is particularly so in the case of communities that have historically been marginalized. For a long time the voices of people of color, immigrants, members of the LGBTQ community, and similarly marginalized groups were listened to less than the voices of the majority. Only fairly recently has society started to draw on the perspective of these groups as a resource toward deeper understanding—a resource that cannot be found outside the lived experience of these communities.

For example, it is clear that certain aspects of the immigrant experience are nearly impossible to know without having undergone them oneself. Much can be surmised, much can be imagined, but there will always be a perspective that is the immigrant's alone. The same is true of other marginalized groups. There are certain elements to being LGBTQ that cannot be known by those who do not identify as such. There are aspects of being Black in America that are likewise understood only by those who have lived this identity. Even between marginalized groups—with their shared understanding of outsider status—certain experiences cannot easily be translated. If this is so, how much harder it is for the majority to fully understand the experience of a minority without the direct input of members of marginalized communities? This question applies to all professional fields—from scientific inquiry to pedagogy. Our own understanding thus is incomplete if we do not try to incorporate the subjective experience of different communities into our broader approach to acquiring knowledge.

In doing so we weave the knowledge that comes from subjective experience into the knowledge that comes from structured methodologies that generate scientific and academic expertise. This form of understanding is based on the principles of logic, reason, and rigorous peer review that have their roots in the ideas of the Enlightenment and the Scientific Revolution. Although the knowledge that emerges from this process can align with our subjective experience and intuition, it does not need to. Indeed, one of the strengths of this approach is that it helps us avoid the missteps that can come with adhering to assumptions simply because they feel right. The scientific process is indifferent to our feelings; its only function is to test our hypotheses and sharpen our thoughts. While lived experience and anecdote can reflect knowledge that is refined over a lifetime—or inherited across generations—the scientific process collapses and intensifies this process of refinement so it can unfold in a controlled setting. This allows us to probe the limits of what we know, test our assumptions, and open the process to collaboration.

Leaning on the epidemiological principles of causation, I would say each of these approaches is necessary but not sufficient for painting an accurate picture of our world and of the forces that shape health. The pursuit of truth—and the maintenance of a liberal public health—is best served by a balance of these two approaches. We need diverse perspectives, the wisdom of inherited cultural knowledge, and the input of community stakeholders to season our expertise, just as surely as we need the methodologies that produce good science. Recent trends that cohere toward such a balance are very much to the good, particularly when they open this process to historically excluded groups. A reoccurring theme of this book is that public health should take a "big tent" approach to its work. We are at our best when we take in the most perspectives in generating our ideas. It is important to engage with community voices in a truly open and welcoming way, avoiding the tokenism that can undermine such efforts. It's not enough simply to pay lip service to the value of individual experience while neglecting the lessons it can convey.

We also should value traditional expertise and the methods that support it. The liberal inheritance of the Enlightenment, whose core is the scientific method, is indispensable. This method, which underlies the generating of expertise, has clearly defined rules that it cannot work without. Other forms of understanding that complement this structure are to be welcomed. Those that undermine or seek to supersede them do no favors for our ability to create knowledge. In balancing these ways of knowing, we can support intellectual inquiry that is at once rigorous and empathetic, technically sound, and motivated by mission and purpose.

SOURCES

"Credentialism and Educational Inflation." Wikipedia. https://en.wikipedia.org/wiki/Credentialism_and_educational_inflation. Published February 13, 2021. Accessed April 29, 2022.

Deb Roy, R. "Decolonise Science–Time to End Another Imperial Era." *Conversation*, April 5, 2018. https://theconversation.com/decolonise-science-time-to-end-another-imperial-era-89189. Accessed April 29, 2022.

Dehaas, J. "Indigenous Ways of Knowing: Magical Thinking and Spirituality by Any One Name." *Quillette*, May 22, 2018. https://quillette.com/2018/05/22/indigenous-ways-knowing-magical-thinking-spirituality-one-name/. Accessed April 29, 2022.

Hennig, C. "'Indigeneer' Combines Scientific Methods and Traditional Indigenous Knowledge." *CBC*, May 9, 2018. https://www.cbc.ca/news/canada/british-columbia/indigeneer-scientific-methods-indigenous-knowledge-1.4655478. Accessed April 29, 2022.

Nichols, T. *The Death of Expertise: The Campaign against Established Knowledge and Why It Matters.* Oxford: Oxford University Press, 2019.

THE AESTHETICS OF A
HEALTHIER WORLD

Public health is as much an aspiration as it is a technical set of skills, tasks, and methods. It is the pursuit of a vision of a healthier world. And this pursuit is more than a technical process; it is an imaginative, creative endeavor. It requires us to radically rethink what the world could be, so that our aspirations may support a future far better than our past. To imagine a radically healthier world is to imagine a world unlike anything we have yet seen. Lacking this frame of reference, in envisioning this future we need to draw on our creative capacities. Along these lines, Leonard Bernstein once said, "Any great work of art . . . revives and readapts time and space, and the measure of its success is the extent to which it makes you an inhabitant of that world, the extent to which it invites you in and lets you breathe its strange, special air."

This speaks to how art, through its aesthetic power, can shape a vision of a different world, one that invites the public to engage with new possibilities for how life could be. Is there any reason the pursuit of health should be less visionary? Bernstein was a master of working within the medium of music to transport listeners to another place. His music for *West Side Story* (with lyrics by Stephen Sondheim), takes listeners to an impressionistic, almost dreamlike version of New York City, which serves as the backdrop for a tale of tragedy and young love. If such care can be taken to craft a fictional world for audiences to enjoy, then public health, which seeks to create a new world in a literal sense, should be just as comfortable working within aesthetic domains as engaging with the more tangible aspects of our field.

Why does this matter for a liberal public health? It matters because an imaginative vision of a healthier world is inseparable from a liberal context where we can think freely about what such a world might look like and then express this vision. This is not to say that art and aesthetics rely exclusively on optimal social and political conditions—creativity can flourish anywhere. Yet it is also true that, outside a liberal context, the aesthetic power of art can suffer. When we are not free to think, we are not free to create. Understanding and expressing the aesthetic vocabulary of a healthier world can support a liberal context for health by keeping at the front of our minds the freedom generated by such a world. Let me take a moment, then, to explore the aesthetics of a healthier world and see how they intersect with a liberal vision for public health.

To start with a basic question, What do we mean by aesthetics? It's easy to think that aesthetic sensibilities simply amount to taste, and in a sense they do. Aesthetic power speaks to our perceptions of beauty, animating our sense of the lovely, the transcendent. This sense is deeply personal. While there is much that we have collectively come to regard as beautiful—nature, for example, and certain works of art—fundamentally, whether something is beautiful lies with the individual beholder. Yet that we perceive beauty at all, regardless of our opinion of particular sights, sounds, and experiences, speaks to a deeper truth about aesthetics: they reflect fundamental values—that of beauty and that of truth. John Keats, one of my favorite Romantic poets, closed his *Ode on a Grecian Urn* with the lines, " 'Beauty is truth, truth beauty,—that is all / Ye know on earth, and all ye need to know.' " This implies that when we experience aesthetic delight, we are relishing an encounter with truth. We love a play or film because it conveys something true about the human experience; we enjoy visual art because it provides a window into a truth about our reality, one we may have missed; we love music for reasons that echo Harlan Howard's definition of country music as "three chords and the truth." We value beauty because we value truth; this is at the core of aesthetic experience. In valuing truth, art and aesthetics have much in common with the science at the heart of public health—the pursuit of truth being core to the liberal inheritance that supports this science.

An aesthetic for a healthier world, then, reflects the truth—about health and about the world that shapes health. The current aesthetic of health does not always fully convey this truth. What are the sights and sounds of health? Likely what first come to mind are images of people exercising— perhaps a workout montage set to music from a film like *Creed*. Then there are young, vibrant faces beaming with fitness. Perhaps we also imagine the logo of some health food or sports drink, or the slogan of a trendy sneaker company. This is an appealing aesthetic, but is it the truth? We in public health know it isn't. It's a slickly packaged presentation of a highly individualized version of the pursuit of health, one that doesn't consider the socioeconomic forces that are, in fact, the overwhelming drivers of health and disease in our society. This aesthetic also, in its focus on youth, leaves out the rest of the life course, suggesting that health is primarily for the young, whereas the truth is that, as populations age, maximizing health increasingly concerns those at the middle and later stage of life. It is also true that a healthier world is indeed one where people live longer, healthier lives, reiterating the importance of an aesthetic that captures the experience of older adults as much as it captures the comings and goings of youth.

In considering an aesthetic for a healthier world, it is also necessary to ask if we are being inclusive enough in our representations of a long, healthy life. A healthier world is one where everyone lives longer, healthier lives regardless of race, sex, gender identity, or sexual orientation. Depicting such a world means more than just featuring people of different backgrounds in our cultural depictions of health. It means declining to traffic in stereotypes of who gets sick and why. It is, of course, true that certain demographic groups feel the burden of certain diseases more acutely; this reality is central to the study of health disparities. But this should be depicted accurately, as a product of foundational socioeconomic forces, rather than as a failing somehow intrinsic to certain groups. It is an unfortunate fact, for example, that for a long time LGBTQ characters were depicted in film, television, and literature as fundamentally tragic, often dying by the end of the story. This was also frequently true of portrayals of biracial characters. The aesthetics of a healthier world would counter these stereotypes, representing these populations to better reflect the truth about their lives. This does not mean the aesthetics of a healthier world should shy away from the tragic aspects of population health, only that depicting this reality should include an accurate view of all who suffer from poor health, rather than focusing on a single stigmatized group.

Finally, the aesthetics of a healthier world should incorporate art that depicts the path from where we are to where we hope to be. To me, one of the most affecting examples of such art has long been Tony Kushner's play *Angels in America: A Gay Fantasia on National Themes*. I remember clearly when I first saw the play, at a time when I was practicing clinical medicine. It felt like a representation in poetry of the prose of reality. The play depicts the darkness of the HIV/AIDS crisis in a way that does not stigmatize its victims, or flinch at depicting the social forces that threatened them, while offering a near-mystical vision of how society might be transformed—indeed, transfigured—into a healthier, more just and inclusive place. The play premiered in the early 1990s, a time when the end of

AIDS and full social equality for the LGBTQ population still seemed far off. Although neither of these goals has yet been fully realized on a global scale, we are far closer than we were when *Angels in America* opened, showing that we can indeed progress toward a vision of a better future first depicted in the aesthetic language of art.

Note that I am not saying we should aspire to create art mainly as a means of making a political or moral case for a specific vision of health. Such motivations can from time to time produce good art, but they can also produce an abundance of well-meaning but aesthetically flat work. Generating art is a fundamentally mysterious process, inspired as much, if not more, by the interior creative vision of the artist as by her external ideological commitments. Producing bad art in the interest of health could arguably be worse for the goal of creating a healthier world than producing no art at all. Instead, public health can inform the aesthetics of a healthier world much the way New York City in the early 1960s informed the Greenwich Village folk music scene that produced Bob Dylan. It can be a place where the currents that shape art meet, creating an aesthetic all its own. To study the forces that shape health from a public health perspective is to intimately engage with the foundational realities of our world, a must for any artist. As we pursue an inclusive vision of a healthier world, our pursuit should include the company of artists, whose talents can help express the human condition as it intersects with the forces that shape health. Their perspective can also sharpen our appreciation of our liberal inheritance, central as it is to supporting a context in which art and artists can thrive.

In addition to creating space for artists in the work of public health, we can also benefit from incorporating the art they create. In preparing presentations, for example, I have often found it very effective to include a piece of art among the charts and graphs I use as visual aids. At various points, references to the work of Shakespeare, the life of the blues musician Blind Willie Johnson, and many other artistic allusions have been helpful in conveying the story of public health.

Health, like art, deals with universal truths about human nature and society. The shared pursuit of these truths reflects a synergy that can enrich our work. An aesthetic for a healthier world combines artistic insight with the rigorous, data-informed perspective of public health. Such an aesthetic, in addition to lending greater beauty to the expression of our ideas—worthwhile for its own sake—can shape an imaginative vision of a liberal public health to inspire hopes for a better future. It can show us what we stand to lose if we abandon our liberal roots and can remind us of the progress ushered in by a liberal engagement with the hard work of creating a better world.

SOURCES

Angels in America (play). Wikipedia. https://en.wikipedia.org/wiki/Angels_in_America. Accessed April 29, 2022.

Creed (film). Wikipedia. https://en.wikipedia.org/wiki/Creed_(film). Accessed April 29, 2022.

Framke, C. "Queer Women Have Been Killed on Television for Decades: Now The 100's Fans Are Fighting Back." *Vox*, March 25, 2016. https://www.vox.com/2016/3/25/11302564/lesbian-deaths-television-trope. Accessed April 29, 2022.

"Harlan Howard: Three Chords and the Truth." Country Music Hall of Fame. https://country musichalloffame.org/content/uploads/2019/05/WM-3-6-Harlan-Howard-Bio.pdf. Accessed April 29, 2022.

Harris, J. "Happy 80th Birthday to Bob Dylan, Rock's Most Prescient Timeless Voice." *Guardian*, May 23, 2021. https://www.theguardian.com/commentisfree/2021/may/23/bob-dylan-80th-birthday-rock. Accessed April 29, 2022.

Johnson, L. A. *A Toolbox for Humanity: More Than 9000 Years of Thought*. Victoria, BC: Trafford, 2004.

Keats, J. "Ode on a Grecian Urn." Poetry Foundation. https://www.poetryfoundation.org/poems/44477/ode-on-a-grecian-urn. Accessed April 29, 2022.

Lee, B. "LGBT Cinema Still Needs More Happy Endings." *Guardian*, October 31, 2018. https://www.theguardian.com/film/commentisfree/2018/oct/31/lgbt-cinema-still-needs-more-happy-endings. Accessed April 29, 2022.

Sablich, J. "From Macdougal Street to 'The Bitter End,' Exploring Bob Dylan's New York." *New York Times*, October 18, 2016. https://www.nytimes.com/2016/10/18/travel/exploring-bob-dylans-greenwich-village-new-york.html. Accessed April 29, 2022.

West Side Story. Wikipedia. https://en.wikipedia.org/wiki/West_Side_Story. Accessed April 29, 2022.

INTELLECTUAL CROSS-TRAINING
TOWARD A HEALTHIER WORLD

One of the ways illiberalism may seem appealing is that it appears to promise greater efficiency. A liberal approach to problems—with its messiness, its airing of different views, and its often slow reasoned analysis—can seem less than nimble in facing the challenges public health engages with. By contrast, an approach that discards liberalism can seem quicker and more decisive—efficient. The classic example in the political realm is the difference between liberal democracy and dictatorship. Liberal democracy can be slow and subject to gridlock, whereas a dictatorship, with all decisions in the hands of one person, can seem far faster and more responsive to the demands of the moment. But do these appearances reflect reality? In the short term, illiberalism can seem a more efficient political model, but in the long term it is often liberal democracy that thrives, adapting to changes while safeguarding the rights of citizens, whereas dictatorship descends into tyranny and falls. This is admittedly an extreme example, but the basic principles—seemingly slow but resilient liberalism versus efficient but brittle totalitarianism—are relevant. Advancing liberalism means appreciating the value of approaches that can seem inefficient in the moment but, when viewed in a broader perspective, are shown to inform a useful—indeed, indispensable—process of human organization. Here, then, are some reflections on how we can cultivate the habits of mind that allow us to see the value of the liberal procedures that, while seeming to meander, are in fact our best route to a healthier world.

Among the things I tried to learn as we navigated the COVID-19 pandemic was how best to learn from inefficiency. Let me explain. It seems to me that when we are at our best as a society, we aspire to efficiency in pursuit of excellence. This pursuit entails looking for ways to maximize our time and resources—a focus on improving skills and finding ways to enhance productivity. In public health, we pursue efficiency with the aim of shaping a healthier world. This lends itself to a particular worldview in which we tend to see events based on the conditions that shape health and our commitment to improving these conditions.

This perspective characterized our response during COVID, both yielding success and disclosing some shortcomings. It allowed us to get much right, helping us provide the public with effective recommendations as we navigated the pandemic. But a fair assessment of our performance would have to concede that we also had some blind spots, areas that fell outside our perspective, exposing the limits of our collective focus. We did not always account for how far partisan politics mediated the way populations engaged with public health recommendations, nor were we always effective at seeing our own biases and realizing how they engendered mistrust among the populations we serve. Instead, we did what we do—focused on the core aims of our field, worked to refine our methods, and proceeded from there. That this focus could occasionally blind us to our lapses into illiberalism reflects the drawbacks of an approach seeking efficiency at all costs.

This suggests that there is more to getting better at our mission of supporting health than pursuing efficiency alone. There is also the richness that comes from the interstices, from seeming inefficiencies, from the detours that ultimately take us to a different, perhaps better, destination than where we thought we were going.

A relevant example is the difference between video conferencing and the in-person interactions we took for granted before the pandemic. At one level, meetings on platforms like Zoom are highly efficient, allowing colleagues to connect without the time and expense of commuting to work. At another level, they can filter out much of the generative energy that comes with meeting in person and bouncing ideas off colleagues in the same physical space. The efficiency of a Zoom call thus is not efficiency in the fullest sense, because it cannot connect us to the unique energy of people gathering together. Gathering in person could indeed seem to be a detour from the efficiency promised by video conferencing, yet it may well bring us more quickly to where we want to go—to ideas that support a healthier world.

Seeking out such apparent detours so as to more effectively reach our goal can seem like a paradox, and perhaps it is one. But it is also a common means of pursuing excellence. Take cross-training. The most prominent examples of cross-training come from the sports world. Elite athletes often cross-train, practicing sports outside their immediate discipline to make more well rounded and ultimately better players. Just as football players may practice ballet, or runners may swim and cycle, we can all benefit from methods of working that expose us to techniques, ideas, and day-to-day interactions we might not have encountered through a narrow focus on only the tasks and experiences that seem to pertain directly to our field.

The uses of what we might call intellectual cross-training include expanding the range of perspectives we bring to generating ideas. In our focus on improving discrete skill sets and applying the perspective of our field to the issues we face (we should continue to do both, even as we broaden our focus), we are liable to miss the richness that comes with taking in new perspectives, new skills, and ideas out of left field. The same is true when we find ourselves trapped in media feedback loops and make no effort to break out of the groupthink they can lead to. If we avoid widening our bandwidth this way, we risk losing this richer sense of the context in which the issues that shape health unfold. A specialized focus can be useful, sharpening our core competencies and deepening our sense of the narrative of public health, but when specialization veers into a narrowness of vision, we can't be fully effective in our pursuit of health. Likewise, neglecting our liberal inheritance can cause our work to lose out on much richness—to say nothing of the intellectual peril of discarding core methodologies.

A lack of the perspective brought by intellectual cross-training may have made it harder to grasp certain aspects of the COVID moment. There was much during the pandemic that we in public health were prepared for—or as prepared as anyone could be in such novel circumstances—but there was also a lot that took many of us by surprise. Such surprises included the high level of public antipathy toward masks, the roots of vaccine hesitancy, the surprisingly strong showing of former president Trump in the election despite his manifest failures at handling the pandemic, and the controversy over the origins of COVID. These issues are difficult to understand fully without a perspective beyond the narrow pursuit of efficiency, mediated by our core biases and preoccupations. What is needed is an expansive approach to health, an openness to diverse perspectives, expressed in random human interactions, freewheeling intellectual curiosity, attention to a wide range of media—some far outside our political and cultural comfort zones—and an embrace of the liberal framework that supports these approaches.

One more point emerges from this perspective. A path that allows us to meander to better ideas may allow us better access to the compassion that comes with seeing more deeply and understanding more fully. The more we embrace detours, the more we can engage with the people living on the streets we might not otherwise have visited. This generates compassion by bringing us into direct contact with individuals and ideas we might otherwise have only heard about secondhand. While efficiency has ample uses, these uses rarely include the digressions that lead us down these unfamiliar streets. To get to a healthier world, we may want to consider paths that twist and turn, allowing the happy accidents, fortuitous encounters, and new perspectives that support a fuller view of health.

SOURCES

Smith, J., and C. Grayhack. "What Is Cross-Training and What Are the Best Activities to Try?" *Runner's World*, September 8, 2021. https://www.runnersworld.com/training /a20827090/16-cross-training-activities-to-try/. Accessed April 29, 2022.

"Why Do Football Players Practice Ballet?" Boss Ballet Barres. https://www.balletbarreson line.com/blogs/news/93291073-why-do-football-players-practice-ballet. Accessed April 29, 2022.

THE INCREDIBLE POTENTIAL
OF NEW TECHNOLOGY

For several years I have been an active participant in the debate over precision medicine. The development of precision medicine reflects our growing capacity to tailor treatments that engage not just with specific diseases, but with the specific physiology of patients, at the genetic level. This opens the door to an array of custom treatments that could revolutionize our ability to leverage emerging technology toward more effectively treating disease. There is much excitement over this potential, and justifiably so.

As it happens, however, I have often found myself feeling a bit misunderstood in these conversations. My point was never that precision medicine cannot do much good. My point was, and is, that we should not let the promise of new technologies distract us from the socioeconomic foundations of health, the forces that decide whether we get sick in the first place. Technology is to be welcomed as long as it is used in concert with this broader focus, with the understanding that even the best technology cannot shape a world that is truly healthy if we do not to shore up the foundations of health.

It is also true that technology can be a powerful support for both liberalism and its alternatives within public health. Technology can create a more inclusive public debate or it can make censorship easier. It can aid the reasoned pursuit of scientific truth or it can amplify shoddy thinking. It can help us retain and sharpen our individual perspectives or it can promote groupthink. Its promise can lead us to see liberal principles as obsolete throwbacks as we move into a utopian techno- future, or it can advance a rebirth of old ideas in new digital spaces. Supporting a liberal public health means reckoning with new technologies and their potential for both good and ill.

Engaging with new technologies is also necessary to ensure that they do not distract us from the fundamental concerns of public health—the socioeconomic conditions we live under. My argument is simply that we should not expect technology to solve all our problems, that we should recognize the deep roots of poor health in our society and address these challenges at their source. Although our technology is formidable, social, economic, and political challenges have created a world that is not as healthy as it could be. This allowed the COVID-19 pandemic to take hold and complicated our efforts to control the virus—whether by hindering vaccine delivery or by maintaining a dysfunctional political status quo that made us far less nimble than was needed in the face of emerging variants.

It is also important that our focus on engaging with the central drivers of health not cause us to devalue the incredible potential of new technologies. From mRNA vaccines, to genomics, to the promise of big data, we are living at a time when new technologies are poised to transform our capacity to support health in ways unprecedented in human history. Technology is a fundamentally positive influence, and innovation in technology has long enriched the work of public health. From simple technologies like hand sanitizer to the use of condoms and PrEP medication to prevent HIV to the use of machine learning and big data in modeling and tracking health behaviors among populations, technology and public health have historically gone hand in hand, to beneficial effect.

So the question is, How can technology best be integrated into an approach to public health that responds to the challenges of the moment while supporting a liberal vision for a changing society? As I answer this, three principles come to mind that could guide our use of technology in the years to come.

First, technology should never be seen as the be-all and end-all of our engagement with health. Even the most effective technologies will not keep us healthy if we do not also engage with the foundations of health. As COVID has shown, we need a balance between foundational engagement and cutting-edge technology if we are to truly progress. We should aspire, always, for this balance in our approach to health.

Second, we should use technology with an eye to eliminating health divides. New technologies, particularly in their early days, are often most accessible to those with the most resources. This can deepen a status quo of health haves and have-nots in which only the rich can reap the benefits of new technologies, while populations with fewer resources lag behind. We already face such a status quo around health, with the socioeconomically vulnerable likeliest to face poor health as a consequence of their material circumstances. This is true in the United States, where men at the bottom of the economic ladder live fifteen years less than their counterparts at the top and women at the bottom live ten years less, and it is true globally, where deep inequities persist on a range of health challenges, from child mortality to infectious diseases like tuberculosis. Exponential change in health technologies could significantly deepen these divides if we do not work to ensure that everyone shares the benefits of innovation, not just the privileged few. If technological development was coupled with a focus on ensuring an equitable distribution of the fruits of innovation, we could do much to ameliorate these divides and create a healthier world.

Finally, we should make an effort to use technology in ways that do not abuse the principles of small-*l* liberalism that underpin a healthy world. As technology allows for ever-greater concentrations of data in the hands of ever-fewer numbers of people and organizations, it is important that these data are not used to undermine fundamental rights. This issue is particularly sensitive when it comes to medical data. When the system of engaging with these data lacks accountability and transparency, it threatens the privacy and well-being of many. Thus new technologies should be accompanied by new norms of conduct concerning the collection and use of data. These norms would ideally be the product of collective decision-making rather than of closed corporate processes, as we work together in the democratic space to create sensible guardrails for the use of new technology.

At the same time, we should take care that our efforts to curb abuses do not veer into censorship or into ideologically motivated constraints on the use of technology. During the COVID moment, we saw the difficulty of striking this balance, as the spread of misinformation on social media posed a real threat to public health. Yet heavy-handed efforts to manage misinformation through, for example, censorship and demonetizing You-Tube videos arguably helped to sow mistrust of the mainstream narrative about the pandemic and to generate skepticism about public health messaging. An example of this was the evolution of the hypothesis that the virus had leaked from a Chinese laboratory. Early in the pandemic this idea was regarded by many as a conspiracy theory, and videos discussing it were often removed from social media. Later the theory gained more mainstream acceptance, and such censorship became less widespread. This reversal was often cited in the online conversation about COVID as an example of the alleged untrustworthiness of public health authorities, big tech, and the media establishment, encouraging the skepticism that would characterize much of the antivaccine movement. Even when they are not used to censor, social media platforms can play a key role in maintaining the media feedback loops that generate groupthink and harden ideological divides.

This situation speaks to the importance of engaging with new technologies guided by the values that have long sustained a liberal society. Free speech, democratic accountability, and a thoughtful, rules-based order have served us well through earlier technologic upheavals, notably the Industrial Revolution. We would do well to continue to adhere to these basic principles as we navigate the challenges and opportunities ahead.

SOURCES

"Child Mortality Rate, 2019." Our World in Data. https://ourworldindata.org/grapher /child-mortality-igme. Accessed April 29, 2022.

Chowkwanyun, M., B. Bayer, and S. Galea. " 'Precision' Public Health—Between Novelty and Hype." *New England Journal of Medicine* 379, no. 15 (2018): 1398–1400.

Flam, F. "Facebook, YouTube Erred in Censoring Covid-19 'Misinformation.' " *Bloomberg*, June 7, 2021. https://www.bloomberg.com/opinion/articles/2021-06-07/facebook -youtube-erred-in-censoring-covid-19-misinformation. Accessed April 29, 2022.

Galea, S. *The Contagion Next Time.* Oxford: Oxford University Press, 2021.

"How Can We Reduce Disparities in Health?" Health Inequality Project. https://health inequality.org. Accessed April 29, 2022.

NCI Scientific Events and Resources. "Will Precision Medicine Improve Public Health?" YouTube. https://www.youtube.com/watch?v=3qjTfpCiT9o. Published June 27, 2016. Accessed April 29, 2022.

Sayers, F. "How Facebook Censored the Lab Leak Theory." *UnHerd*, May 31, 2021. https:// unherd.com/2021/05/how-facebook-censored-the-lab-leak-theory/. Accessed April 29, 2022.

Stephens, B. "Media Groupthink and the Lab-Leak Theory." *New York Times*, May 31, 2021. https://www.nytimes.com/2021/05/31/opinion/media-lab-leak-theory.html. Accessed April 29, 2022.

THE CONSENT OF THE GOVERNED

During the pandemic, government at the local and national level was criticized for failures in mitigating COVID-19 and in addressing any number of the problems we collectively face. Such criticism is often warranted, even helpful. Power needs accountability so it can be used most effectively to support the common good. However, in much of this criticism there was an implicit belief that people in positions of leadership have more power to sway events than they actually do have. We seem to believe that somewhere there is a magic wand that can solve our problems, and that only some kind of obstinacy stops those in power from waving it.

Public health is not immune to this belief. We often fault those in power for doing less than we think they are capable of in the face of crisis. And we can find ourselves perhaps too eager to align with those in power for just this reason—we think they are best positioned to make the changes we want to see. This can lead us to illiberal behavior as pursuing proximity to power causes us to neglect our core principles. It also suggests comfort with modes of leadership that concentrate power in the hands of an "effective" few, far from the democratic messiness of the many. This too reflects the illiberalism that has characterized our field at times in recent years.

It's important to note here that belief in a vision of power where leaders are free to do more or less whatever they like does not reflect the most common reality of leadership. That belief perhaps betrays our lack of understanding of how far leaders' capacity to do, well, anything depends on us—on the consent of the governed. In my writing, I have found myself returning to a telling quotation from Abraham Lincoln: "Public sentiment is everything. With public sentiment, nothing can fail; without it, nothing can succeed." The power of public opinion is such that even a relatively low level of public engagement can be enough to reshape society. Research has suggested, for example, that it takes about 3.5 percent of a population actively engaging in political protests to bring about real political change.

Given this power, if the public withholds its consent from a given measure, governments face a steep climb toward its successful implementation. It does not matter how much good the measure might do; without the consent of the governed, it cannot take effect to any significant degree. It can look as if this ineffectiveness is solely the fault of incompetent leadership, when leadership may be doing all it can if public consent is withheld.

This consent is more than just the linchpin of effective policy. It is arguably the cornerstone of the entire philosophy of liberal governance refined during the Enlightenment, notably by the political philosopher John Locke, which forms the basis for our political system in the United States. According to Locke, the basis for this consent was the understanding that the people would willingly surrender some of their rights to the government in exchange for that government's safeguarding life, liberty, property rights, and the public good. This arrangement was regarded as provisional, reserving to the people the right to resist any government that did not uphold the social contract.

We see reflections of this contract throughout our society. Take traffic laws, in which we surrender to these laws our freedom to navigate the open road at whatever speed we like, with the understanding that doing so will keep us and those around us safer. The power of this social contract is shown in the way we abide by it even without heavy-handed enforcement mechanisms. How often, for example, do you sit at a stoplight at night, with no one around? Why don't you speed through it? The answer is likely, in part, because you believe that consenting to the rules is better for all of us, that the system of regulations the stoplight represents helps support a better, healthier world in clearly tangible ways.

But what if we quit believing this? What happens when, rightly or wrongly, we no longer trust those with power to uphold their end of the social contract? We need not look far for answers—we've seen what happened among those who resisted COVID vaccination. Large numbers of people withheld their consent; not only that, they withheld it on an issue where their consent could have made the difference between life and death. They chose, it might be said, to speed through traffic lights, despite the risk and the urgings of the common good. Why?

There are three main reasons, and understanding them is a key part of our learning that emerges from the COVID pandemic. The first reason is lack of trust. Many people simply don't believe the government has their best interests at heart. Examples of political dishonesty, both real and imagined, have exacerbated this belief. Much of the most vocal distrust of vaccines was concentrated on the political right. However, it is worth remembering that, early in the pandemic, some on the political left expressed skepticism about any vaccine developed under the Trump administration, given the administration's record of false and misleading statements. This reflects the way distrust can spread across the political spectrum, and it shows that leaders should be wary of adding to it by willfully misleading behavior.

This leads to a second threat to the integrity of the social contract: the cynical exploitation of societal divisions by political actors. Implicit in the social contract between the people and the government is the understanding that both parties will attempt to behave responsibly, guided by reason and a pragmatic concern for the public good. It is a delicate balance, which is always vulnerable to those who would exploit the status quo to gain personal power. Societal divisions have always existed, but a responsible leader, working within the liberal order, will aim to bridge these divides, or at least not to inflame them. Unfortunately, some will choose to do the opposite, calculating that the path of the demagogue is a quicker route to prominence than that of the measured consensus builder. There is a long tradition of such figures in the United States, and they have thrived in recent years, with the internet making it easier than ever to cultivate and monetize large followings based on whatever compels attention, even at the expense of the public good. Such figures further polarize the spread of information, making it increasingly difficult to know who or what to believe.

In doing so, these figures often make use of misinformation. This is the third key challenge to maintaining the consent of the governed. If a debate is polluted by misinformation, it does not matter how well reasoned the logic of leadership is, it will always face the obstacle of falsehoods masquerading as facts. For misinformation to thrive requires two key factors: first, it needs figures unscrupulous enough disseminate it. Second, it requires that established authorities have indeed occasionally been dishonest or, at least, inconsistent in their messaging. Such failures open the door to those who say that truth is relative, or that the occasional missteps of those in positions of authority mean that nothing they say should be trusted.

What do these challenges to the social contract, and to the consent of the governed, teach us about how we should talk about health to encourage healthy behaviors in the years to come?

Chiefly, they teach us the importance of trust. For populations to consent to measures meant to improve public health, they must trust the people who are recommending them. For those of us trying to promote these measures, this means, frankly, being trustworthy. This does not just mean not telling lies; it also means not giving the appearance of telling lies by being evasive, unclear, or inconsistent in our communication. During COVID, for example, it could sometimes seem that some of us used our mandate to follow the data as a crutch for inconsistent communication. If we contradicted ourselves, we could simply say we did so because the data changed. Now, sometimes the data really did change. Other times, however, it did not, but perhaps the political or social incentives had changed, causing us to reverse a position or walk back previous statements. Regardless of whether we were justified in claiming changing data as the reason for these reversals, such behavior can seem dishonest—illiberal—eroding the consent we rely on for our message to resonate.

The challenges of recent years also teach us the importance of self-evaluation, to ensure that we are not ourselves using the conditions of crisis to advance our power. This is particularly crucial given that most people who join the work of public health do so with good intentions. When they seek power, it is not for its own sake, but to support health. Yet our good intentions can make it harder for us to see when we have fallen short of our ideals and may indeed need to rethink our relation to power. To behave in ways that align with the consent of the governed, then, we must engage in continual self-reflection, to ensure that our uses of power are never reminiscent of the demagogues that recent years have produced.

At core, supporting a social contract that relies on the consent of the governed means giving priority to truthful engagement with the needs and perspectives of the populations we serve—something that should be guiding our efforts at all times. Encouraging healthy behaviors requires transparency about why these behaviors are necessary, and the understanding that the public's buy-in is always provisional and should not be taken for granted or abused. For the public to uphold their end of the contract, we must uphold ours, working collaboratively and respectfully within a liberal framework toward a healthier world for all.

SOURCES

Lincoln, A. "II: In the First Debate with Douglas." Bartleby. https://www.bartleby.com/268 /9/23.html. Accessed April 29, 2022.

"Locke's Political Philosophy." *Stanford Encyclopedia of Philosophy*. https://plato.stanford .edu/entries/locke-political/. Published November 9, 2005. Updated October 6, 2020. Accessed April 29, 2022.

Robson, D. "The '3.5% Rule': How a Small Minority Can Change the World." BBC, May 13, 2019. https://www.bbc.com/future/article/20190513-it-only-takes-35-of-people-to -change-the-world. Accessed April 29, 2022.

Satter, R. "Kamala Harris Says Trump Not Credible on Possible COVID-19 Vaccine." *Reuters*, September 15, 2020. https://www.reuters.com/article/health-coronavirus-usa -politics/kamala-harris-says-trump-not-credible-on-possible-covid-19-vaccine-idUS KBN25X01L. Accessed April 29, 2022.

SPENDING SMARTER

I have long argued that it's not enough simply to pour money into what we think is supporting health if those funds don't properly target what truly shores up the foundations of health in our society. The classic example is our investment in health care. The United States invests more in health care than any other country in the world, yet our health is mediocre compared with that of peer nations. This is the very definition of an investment that doesn't pay off as fully as it should. In talks I give, I often compare this to investing in a smartphone. Imagine if smartphones were far more expensive in the United States than in other countries yet were slower and held less data than smartphones one can buy overseas. Would we accept this? I suggest we would not. Yet we accept this disparity when it comes to health. This situation has created a status quo that has made us, collectively, less healthy than we could and should be. This preventable poor health set us up to fail during COVID-19.

The pandemic was a warning: unless we spend smarter on health, we will not be as healthy as we could be, leaving us vulnerable to future pandemics. It will also leave us vulnerable to illiberalism. A healthy society is generally less likely to experience the desperation, cynicism, and despair that can lead to an embrace of illiberalism in politics, institutions, and society. We cannot build a healthy society if our spending is misaligned with the actual causes of our health status. This issue is particularly salient at present, when we are poised to spend more than ever on what we believe matters most for health. The crisis of COVID created new avenues at the federal level for spending the money we should be investing in health. We have seen an influx of attention and resources directed toward mitigating the effects of the pandemic. The COVID-era federal stimulus is an example of the kind of investment that, if properly directed toward the core drivers of health, could do much to shape a healthier country. As we see new openings for such investment, now is an excellent time to reflect on how we currently spend on health, and on how we can do so more effectively, toward supporting a healthy society where liberalism retains its appeal.

It seems helpful to begin by focusing on some principles that can guide our investment going forward. These principles have long been central to the work of population health science; my colleague Katherine Keyes and I engaged with them in our 2016 book on the subject.

UNDERSTANDING THAT DISEASES ARE MULTILEVEL AND GENERATED OVER TIME

At present, much of our health investment reflects a view of health that is confined to the narrow period when it gives way to disease. We tend to think of sickness as episodes in our life, moments when, feeling bad, we go to the doctor and she tries to cure us. But this is not an accurate view of what health really is. Health is an emergent property of our whole life and the conditions that shape it. Perhaps, for example, we have heart disease. While it may seem like an unfortunate episode in our life, looking at the full picture of health can help us see that the disease reflects multiple layers of influence over an extended period, which gradually laid the groundwork for disease. Heart disease is often a consequence of obesity, which is in turn a consequence of a range of complex factors that influence our health over the long run. These factors include the accessibility (or lack) of nutritious foods in our neighborhoods, the ingredients we subsidize at the federal level (often unhealthy processed food), and norms around portion sizes in restaurants. The intersection of these forces over time is what truly shapes health and is where our investment, and intervention, should be focused. We could, for example, invest in subsidizing healthier foods and in building neighborhoods where nutritious options are easily accessible. We could reduce portion sizes and even tax sugary drinks, using the funds we raise to invest even more in the foundational drivers of health. All these doors begin to open once we see the full range of factors that shape health.

MAINTAINING FOCUS ON THE UBIQUITOUS FORCES THAT MATTER MOST FOR HEALTH

Our health investment currently is deep but narrow. It is deep in the sense that it is seemingly bottomless in terms of the money we are willing to spend; it is narrow in that the vast majority of these funds goes to doctors, medicines, and treatments. The forces that truly shape health, however, are as broad as they are ubiquitous. They are the air we breathe, the food we eat, the water we drink, the places where we live, work, and play, our political systems, how far our society supports social and economic justice, and more. For our spending to make an impact, it must address these ubiquitous conditions. We need to broaden what we think of as health spending, to ensure that our investment engages with the forces that shape health.

KNOWING THAT PREVENTION IS MORE COST-EFFECTIVE THAN CURE

Benjamin Franklin said that an ounce of prevention is worth a pound of cure. When we invest in creating a context where disease does not emerge, we help to prove his adage correct. By prevention, I do not mean exclusively preventive care. I mean the prevention that comes with shaping a world where disease does not take hold. In that world we could forestall the astronomical costs imposed on us by sicknesses that emerge from a society that is not optimized for health. For example, from 2000 to 2002, the truth antismoking campaign spent about $324 million to help prevent youth smoking. Later analysis found that the campaign helped save society nearly $1.9 billion in estimated medical costs as of 2009. Spending smarter on health means investing in prevention, to save money in the long run as well as—most important—saving lives.

ACCEPTING THAT WHAT MATTERS FOR EQUITY MAY NOT BE THE SAME AS WHAT MATTERS MOST FOR HEALTH OVERALL

In recent years there has been increased focus within public health on the pursuit of equity. This is reflected in efforts to calibrate systems to produce an equality of outcomes, rather than to achieve the baseline of simple equality, which aspires to equality of opportunity alone. The pursuit of equity has led to engaging with the foundational drivers of health, optimizing them to bring society closer to equality of outcomes. As we invest in this pursuit, we should be mindful that what is good for equity may conflict with what is good for health overall. For example, a pillar of investing in a healthy world is education. Access to quality education is among the foundational drivers of the capacity to live a healthy life. If health and disease are indeed multilevel and shaped over time, education spending is one of the smartest investments we can make in the long-term health of populations. In the United States we have seen much attention paid to gifted programs for younger students. Because minority students are not always proportionately represented in these programs, there has been a push to abolish them entirely, in the interests of equity. As the debate over these programs continues, this strikes me as a case where the pursuit of equity may indeed complicate our broader aim of investing more effectively in a healthier world. It is, of course, possible to make the case that ending these programs serves efforts to ultimately broaden access to education, but the controversy nevertheless demonstrates that our aspirations toward equity can at times run counter to what matters most for health overall, and we should be mindful of this. We should take particular care that our efforts to move beyond mere equality in pursuit of equity do not cause us to turn in an illiberal direction, discarding the safeguards that support the former in our zeal to get to the latter.

Fundamentally, these principles are meant to help construct a better approach to our investment in health. The crisis of COVID did much to broaden our thinking about such investment. At the federal level we saw a growing understanding that investing in the material resources of people's lives *is* investing in health. The pandemic also showed us that the larger context of our lives is key to our health, as our experience of COVID was deeply shaped by the conditions around us, which influenced both our physical and our mental health. This experience only added to the importance of spending smarter on health, as standards shifted about the level of federal investment deemed politically feasible. If we invest wisely, the results could be transformative, supporting a society that aligns with a liberal vision of health. If we misinvest, however, we risk squandering the chance to apply the hard lessons of the COVID moment, and of our long-standing mediocre health, to the project of shaping a better world.

SOURCES

Galea, S. "A Good Education—the Best Prevention?" Boston University School of Public Health. https://www.bu.edu/sph/news/articles/2016/a-good-education-the-best-prevention/. Published May 8, 2016. Accessed April 29, 2022.

Holtgrave, D. R., K. A. Wunderink, D. M. Vallone, and C. G. Healton. "Cost-Utility Analysis of the National Truth Campaign to Prevent Youth Smoking." *American Journal of Preventive Medicine* 36, no. 5 (2009): 385–88.

"How Does the U.S. Healthcare System Compare to Other Countries?" Peter G. Peterson
    Foundation. https://www.pgpf.org/blog/2020/07/how-does-the-us-healthcare-system
    -compare-to-other-countries. Published July 14, 2020. Accessed April 29, 2022.

Keyes, K. M., and S. Galea. *Population Health Science*. Oxford: Oxford University Press,
    2016.

Lee, J., and C. Siemaszko. "New York City to Phase Out Gifted and Talented Public School
    Programs That Critics Call Racist." *NBC News*, October 8, 2021. https://www.nbcnews
    .com/news/us-news/new-york-city-phase-out-gifted-talented-public-school-programs
    -n1281134. Accessed April 29, 2022.

Oaklander, M. "Many Foods Subsidized by the Government Are Unhealthy." *Time*, July 5,
    2016. https://time.com/4393109/food-subsidies-obesity/. Accessed April 29, 2022.

"Ounce of Prevention, Pound of Cure." University of Cambridge. https://www.cam.ac.uk
    /research/news/ounce-of-prevention-pound-of-cure. Published October 9, 2012.
    Accessed April 29, 2022.

Siegel, R. "What's in Congress's $1.9 Trillion Covid Bill: Checks, Unemployment, Insurance
    and More." *Washington Post*, March 10, 2021. https://www.washingtonpost.com/business
    /2021/03/10/what-is-in-the-stimulus/. Accessed April 29, 2022.

A POPULIST PUBLIC HEALTH

Ever since roughly 2015, much has been written about populism. The catalyst for this was three political events occurring within months of each other. First there was the rise of Donald Trump and Bernie Sanders in the presidential primaries of 2015–16. Each in his own way—one from the political right and one from the political left—seemed to speak to the concerns of working-class Americans who felt marginalized by globalization and what they perceived as the misrule of social and economic elites. Sanders addressed this by calling for an ambitious program of redistributive economic policies to level a playing field that had long been uneven. Trump's argument, too, was partially economic, embracing protectionist trade policies and hostility to NAFTA. He was also—rhetorically, at least (his policies in office would prove another matter)—more sympathetic to the existing welfare state than many Republican candidates of the past. But his populism was tinged with illiberalism and had racist and xenophobic overtones, which both fueled his political ascent and arguably poisoned the well of our public discourse in ways we have not yet recovered from. Largely because of Trump, much of the discourse around populism was primed to view the phenomenon as, on the whole, a negative influence—crude, anti-intellectual, and even racist. This view was seemingly confirmed in the months before the presidential election, when voters in the United Kingdom chose to leave the European Union. Many saw this move as motivated by reaction to high levels of immigration and by hostility toward the bureaucratic elite running the EU. Widespread fear of the potential economic and political ramifications of the Brexit vote meant it would do no favors for populism's reputation, at least among those not part of the demographic that had already proved receptive to a populist message. Then there was the rise of populist far-right parties throughout Europe. This too cast populism in a negative light and helped it become, for many, synonymous with far-right politics in general.

The specter of a resurgent right-wing populism also did much to instigate illiberalism in public health. As I've written in previous chapters, the
clear and present threat of this form of populism seemed to justify emergency measures within our field, even when such measures tilted into illiberalism. These measures encouraged greater politicizing of public health
as we became more openly aligned with progressivism generally and the
Democratic Party specifically. I am not here to argue that the threat was
overblown, or that our reaction to it was not understandable. I am saying
that we must understand populism—its philosophy and its appeal—if we
are to counter it or, better yet, co-opt it toward advancing a liberal vision
of a healthier world.

What, then, is populism? In today's world the word has become all
but synonymous with its worst aspects. It is easy to forget that, freed of
its contemporary baggage, populism can mean simply standing with the
socioeconomically marginalized, giving priority to their concerns over
the interests of the powerful. The trouble we have seen is the wedding of
populist rhetoric to policies that often favor the very elites that the faux-
populist rails against—and that disadvantage the dispossessed. But just
because the populist idiom can be vulnerable to corruption does not mean
it should be ceded to its worst practitioners. Indeed, public health owes
much to populism, to a defense of common interests against the preroga-
tives of the powerful elite. A classic example is smoking. For a long time,
cigarette companies monopolized public opinion about their product—a
product that caused tremendous harm to the health of populations. These
companies used slick advertising to sustain an image of smoking as glam-
orous, even healthy. When it became clear, through the 1964 US surgeon
general's report, that smoking was in fact deadly, public health found itself
in the position of the populist, working against corporate interests to stand
up for the well-being of the less powerful. Remember that we waged a
successful campaign against smoking by working within a classically liberal framework. We argued, we persuaded, we led with the truth, and
progress followed. Even in the face of a seemingly unbeatable opponent,
the well-funded smoking industry, we were able to win within the rules
of the liberal game. This is perhaps a lesson for us as we engage with new,
seemingly invulnerable foes. We need not become like those we oppose
in order to win in the marketplace of ideas.

Public health has also historically been interlinked with populist reform movements, notably those of the Progressive Era, in which reformers
stood against entrenched interests to argue for worker protections and

better living conditions in cities. As public health has deepened its focus on improving the material conditions of people's lives as a means of supporting population health, it remains aligned with the classic populist position, arguing on behalf of the marginalized, often facing pushback from powerful interests that benefit from a broken status quo. Given this history, it seems premature and counterproductive to let populism be defined solely by its post-2015 character. This is particularly true after the experience of COVID-19. The polarizing of seemingly every aspect of the pandemic has, for many, led to identifying public health with a caricature of finger-wagging elites in media, government, and academia. This has eroded the trust we rely on to effectively engage with the public and promote health. With this in mind, I would argue that now is the time for a public health that has reengaged with its populist roots.

What would a populist public health look like? First, it would be about people. There is much about the work of public health that can distract us from this core focus. Developing ideas, pursuing science, raising and managing funds, implementing solutions—all are part of our work, and this is all to the good. But we must never forget that these achievements are meant to serve our central aim: improving the health of populations—of people. This work should always be our central aim. Such an aim can also support a liberal vision of public health. When we are centrally concerned with people—as individuals rather than as abstractions—it becomes difficult to deny them the basic rights that liberalism exists to safeguard. When we see people—even our political opponents—as individuals, it becomes harder to censor them and easier to treat them with civility and respect.

Second, a populist public health does not shy away from criticizing power structures that keep in place a status quo that is harmful to health. This is not to say, of course, that we should pick fights. Nor does it mean we should attempt to dismantle (as opposed to reform) systems just because they don't always produce optimal outcomes. We must simply accept the reality that the conditions that shape health are often defined by opposing interests. When one of these interests is a powerful entity acting in ways that undermine health and the other is a less powerful entity whose health is being threatened, we should not equivocate about whose side we are on. This includes criticizing public health itself when its actions are illiberal or in any way run counter to the interests of the populations we serve. This gives us a perspective from which to pursue reform through reason, always respecting the basic societal structures that allow us to air disagreements with civility. Along these lines, we should also work to ensure that the partisan divides of the moment do not cloud our view of who stands on the side of health and who does not. The emotions of the moment make it tempting to feel that anyone who is part of our political in-group is beyond criticism and that anyone in a political out-group is indisputably aligned against our interests. We need to question these assumptions if we are to maintain an accurate view of who really has the best interests of health at heart.

Finally, pursuing a populist public health requires us to rethink our reflexive wariness about populism in general, to advance a more constructive vision of it. There is a reason populism has long been a potent political force: at its best, it speaks to the real needs of people, particularly those who have found themselves voiceless in the public debate. It is even worth revisiting more recent examples of populism to ask ourselves if, beneath its darker elements, it spoke to any legitimate grievances. This reflects another core motivation for pursuing a populist public health: if we don't address such grievances, others will—others who may not be acting in good faith with an eye toward shaping a better world. I've found myself haunted by the title of a 2019 piece by David Frum in the *Atlantic*, "If Liberals Won't Enforce Borders, Fascists Will." It argues for a humane, pragmatic border policy as a means of forestalling a more xenophobic, abusive approach to the issue by those who would co-opt it for destructive political ends. The same goes for populism. A healthful populism can do much to create a healthier world. An unhealthful populism can actively make the world sicker by dividing people and empowering the kind of political figures and movements that do no favors for the work of public health. We need a healthful populism in order to deal with issues within a liberal framework, or we risk ceding them to others who pursue an approach not constrained by the liberal guardrails that support a healthy world.

Public health's central mission is to care for the health of populations, with particular concern for the marginalized and vulnerable. Throughout our history, we have pursued this mission by aligning ourselves with the interests of these groups when they faced challenges. If we are indeed in a populist moment, we should not let that moment be defined by those who use the appearance of populism to mask polices that would harm our constituencies. A populist public health can step into this breach to advance a vision of a better world by speaking to the needs of those who stand to inherit our success or failure in creating it. At the same time, we can work to build bridges between those with power and those with less. Rather than advance a divisive populism, we can promote a populism that helps societies better cohere toward the common good. In a moment with much at stake for health, by rediscovering our populist roots, public health can become an even more effective force for good.

SOURCES

"2016 Presidential Candidates on Federal Assistance Programs." Ballotpedia. https://ballot
    pedia.org/2016_presidential_candidates_on_federal_assistance_programs. Accessed
    April 29, 2022.

Baldini, G., E. Bressanelli, and S. Gianfreda. "Taking Back Control? Brexit, Sovereignism
    and Populism in Westminster (2015–17)." *European Politics and Society* 21, no. 2 (2019):
    219–34.

"Brexit." *Guardian*. https://www.theguardian.com/politics/eu-referendum. Accessed April 29,
    2022.

Frum, D. "If Liberals Won't Enforce Borders, Fascists Will." *Atlantic*, April 2019. https://
    www.theatlantic.com/magazine/archive/2019/04/david-frum-how-much-immigration
    -is-too-much/583252/. Accessed April 29, 2022.

Galea, S. "A Case against Moralism in Public Health." *Healthiest Goldfish* (blog), February 12,
    2021. https://sandrogalea.substack.com/p/a-case-against-moralism-in-public. Accessed
    April 29, 2022.

Gillespie, P. "Trump Hammers America's 'Worst Trade Deal.'" *CNN Business*, September 27,
    2016. https://money.cnn.com/2016/09/27/news/economy/donald-trump-nafta-hillary
    -clinton-debate/. Accessed April 29, 2022.

"History of the Surgeon General's Reports on Smoking and Health." Centers for Disease
    Control and Prevention. https://www.cdc.gov/tobacco/data_statistics/sgr/history
    /index.htm. Updated October 19, 2021. Accessed April 29, 2022.

Katty, K. "US Election 2016: The Trump Protectionist Party." *BBC*, March 24, 2016. https://
    www.bbc.com/news/election-us-2016-35836102. Accessed April 29, 2022.

Liasson, M. "Nativism and Economic Anxiety Fuel Trump's Populist Appeal." *NPR*, Sep-
    tember 4, 2015. https://www.npr.org/sections/itsallpolitics/2015/09/04/437443401
    /populist-movement-reflected-in-campaigns-of-sanders-and-trump. Accessed April 29,
    2022.

Packer, G. "The Populists." *New Yorker*, August 30, 2015. https://www.newyorker.com/mag
    azine/2015/09/07/the-populists. Accessed April 29, 2022.

Prokop, A. "Bernie Sanders 2016: A Primer." *Vox*, October 12, 2015. https://www.vox.com
    /2015/7/28/18093566/bernie-sanders-issues-policies. Accessed April 29, 2022.

"Public Health in the Progressive Era." Oregon Health and Science University. https://www
    .ohsu.edu/historical-collections-archives/public-health-progressive-era. Accessed
    April 29, 2022.

Rosenbaum, D., and E. Neuberger. "President's 2021 Budget Would Cut Food Assistance
    for Millions and Radically Restructure SNAP." Center on Budget and Policy Priorities.
    https://www.cbpp.org/research/food-assistance/presidents-2021-budget-would-cut
    -food-assistance-for-millions-and. Published February 18, 2020. Accessed April 29, 2022.

IN PRAISE OF OBJECTIVE REALITY

We are living, we are often told, in a post-truth moment. The landscape of thoughts and ideas is now seeded with opinions that have little connection with objective reality. On the political right this includes the belief that Donald Trump won the 2020 presidential election despite the electoral math and the repeated failure of his legal challenges. On the political left this disjunction is reflected in a tendency to give personal truths based on identity priority over the reality of a given situation—a tendency captured, for example, by the Black Lives Matter statement defending actor Jussie Smollett despite evidence that he fabricated a racist attack on himself and lied to police about it. Core to these beliefs is the way they are embedded within broader worldviews, narratives embraced by segments of the population with such fervor that anything seeming to contradict them is simply ignored, regardless of the facts. So President Trump won the election because President Trump cannot lose, and Jussie Smollett cannot be guilty because his case was investigated by police and police always lie.

The emergence of a post-truth moment matters for public health for two key reasons. First, the work of public health is fundamentally pursuing truth and conveying that truth to others. If we choose narrative over facts, accepting a worldview that is not based on objective reality, we risk compromising our work and the healthier world we aspire to build. We also risk losing the public trust that our efforts depend on. Second, a liberal worldview is predicated on a grounding in solid truth, even as we recognize that our understanding of truth is subjective and influenced by our biases. When feeling overrides truth in the public square, it opens the door to abuses and an eroding of the small-*l* liberal norms that help sustain our society. Indeed, veering from the pursuit of truth can be seen as by definition illiberal, committed as liberalism is to the objective understanding of reality.

We should remember, always, that a society based on truth—and, indeed, on liberalism—is a society that is working against the current of human nature. It is difficult to keep truth in view, and far easier to let our vision be clouded by biases. Yet reality is powerful and tends to win out, coming to the fore as our illusions and preferred narratives fade. This can happen quickly or it can take a long time, but it is difficult to recall a case where it did not happen eventually. Given the resilience of reality, it is clearly counterproductive to resist engaging with the truth, however comforting our preferred narratives and illusions may be. Ultimately, shaping a healthier world means first seeing the world as it is, in all its paradigm-disrupting messiness. We can then work to build a better world with our eyes open.

How can we ensure that we remain engaged with objective reality in a moment when so much can distract us from it? First, we can encourage numerous voices in the public conversation. In isolation, it becomes easy for us to feel we have the world figured out. We get comfortable in our echo chambers and rarely venture beyond the confines of our long-standing assumptions. Only by hearing from many different perspectives we can see beyond our biases. It can be hard to differentiate between the world as it is and the narratives we choose to believe; engaging with other perspectives can help us discern what is true and what is false by questioning our assumptions and forcing us to think differently about the issues we face. This means rejecting any approach to core issues that tries to censor or drown out opposing views. Such efforts, when they are successful, threaten to blind us to the varying perspectives that are core to widening our field of vision on the issues that shape health.

Second, we need to use our engagement with different perspectives to stress-test our ideas. There are few better ways to determine whether an idea truly reflects reality than to engage with others who are disinclined to believe it. If, for example, climate science can convince a climate change skeptic that global warming poses a threat, this strongly suggests that taking climate change seriously reflects reality. Another example of this stress-testing of ideas is the peer review that is so fundamental to the scientific method. When we open our ideas to criticism and the risk of being disproved, they may emerge stronger. The proliferation of narrative over facts shows how difficult it can be to see beyond our own blind spots. Embracing the marketplace of ideas, in all its occasional raucousness, can free us from seeing the world only through our own eyes. It is true, of course, that some people are so entrenched within their biases that no evidence can persuade them to look beyond their ideological bubbles. Even so, engaging with different perspectives can serve as an intellectual whetstone, sharpening our ideas and revealing where our biases serve us poorly.

Third, we should celebrate the dispassionate pursuit of truth and recognize when narratives threaten to distract us from it. At present we place a premium on individual, subjective truth, often above the inconvenient facts that can complicate narratives. It may be time to rethink how far we as a culture do this. We cannot always be dispassionate in our pursuit of truth—indeed, doing so runs against our deep human impulse to see the world from our own unique perspective. What we can do, however, is decide collectively to celebrate a pursuit of truth informed, as much as possible, by evidence and empiricism. This means resisting narratives that may feel right but are disproved by a preponderance of evidence. Consider vaccine hesitancy. Much of the resistance to vaccines is instigated by a broader skepticism of institutional authority in general, a skepticism that, it must be said, is often warranted. Authority figures do get many things wrong, and they do obfuscate and lie. There have been examples of this throughout the pandemic, on both the left and the right, as individuals and institutions have tilted toward an illiberal engagement with issues. This has prompted a narrative that authority figures are always to be distrusted, including when they say vaccines are safe and effective. But during COVID-19 the data did not support this. Rather, they told us that COVID vaccines were our best chance for avoiding serious complications from the virus. However, the antiauthority, antivaccine narrative was embraced so strongly, particularly on the political right, that even former president Trump encountered pushback when he touted the benefits of vaccines and boosters. On the left, a narrative that encouraged strict COVID mitigation measures led to choices about the pandemic that at times ignored the science in favor of political signaling.

In both examples we see how embracing narrative over facts can be encouraged by our willingness to celebrate stories that seem to support certain subjective truths even in the face of complicating data. Choosing objective reality means rethinking our acceptance of such narratives when they come at the expense of truth. We cannot always know what is true, but we can choose, as a society, to prefer difficult facts over comforting stories that support our existing worldview. In doing so we acknowledge that in the end only truth can support a healthier world. While narrative is an effective, even indispensable, means of conveying the story of health, it is at its best in the service of truth. When we bend truth to serve a narrative, even in pursuit of laudable goals, we build our house on sand, only to have it upended when reality reasserts itself, as reality always does. It is far better, then, to pursue the truth wherever it leads, confident that its ultimate destination is the healthier world we seek.

SOURCES

"Breaking Points: Trump Mocks Anti-vaxxers, Touts MAGA Vaccine Victory." Breaking Points with Krystal and Saagar (video). YouTube. https://www.youtube.com/watch?v =Qj5NOVJMwzk. Published December 21, 2021. Accessed April 29, 2022.

Cummings, W., J. Garrison, and J. Sergent. "By the Numbers: President Donald Trump's Failed Efforts to Overturn the Election." *USA Today*, January 6, 2021. https://www .usatoday.com/in-depth/news/politics/elections/2021/01/06/trumps-failed-efforts -overturn-election-numbers/4130307001/. Accessed April 29, 2022.

Green, E. "The Liberals Who Can't Quit Lockdown." *Atlantic*, May 4, 2021. https://www .theatlantic.com/politics/archive/2021/05/liberals-covid-19-science-denial-lockdown /618780/. Accessed April 29, 2022.

Luxemburg, R. Rosa Luxemburg Quotes. Goodreads. https://www.goodreads.com/author /quotes/25616.Rosa_Luxemburg. Accessed April 29, 2022.

"Post-truth Politics." Wikipedia. https://en.wikipedia.org/wiki/Post-truth_politics. Accessed April 29, 2022.

"Statement regarding the Ongoing Trial of Jussie Smollett." Black Lives Matter. https:// blacklivesmatter.com/statement-regarding-the-ongoing-trial-of-jussie-smollett/. Published December 7, 2021. Accessed April 29, 2022.

THE NEXT GENERATION:
THE KIDS ARE (PROBABLY)
ALL RIGHT

The children now love luxury; they have bad manners, contempt for authority; they show disrespect for elders and love chatter in place of exercise. Children are now tyrants, not the servants of their households. They no longer rise when elders enter the room. They contradict their parents, chatter before company, gobble up dainties at the table, cross their legs, and tyrannize their teachers.

So (allegedly) said Socrates. If the attribution is correct, it appears that even the ancients took part in the time-honored tradition of complaining about the young. What is perhaps most striking about Socrates's complaint is how modern it sounds. His accusations—that the young lack manners, disrespect their elders, talk foolishly, and love luxury (as opposed to honest hard work, presumably)—could well have been said by any older person today, perhaps while shooing the young off the proverbial lawn.

Consider, for example, common criticisms of Millennials and Generation Z—the age cohorts born in the 1980s, 1990s, and early 2000s. They have been accused of entitlement, oversensitivity, and lack of a robust work ethic. These accusations are variations on old themes. It is perhaps as inevitable as the changing seasons that generations eventually grow up, look at the young, and ask, Are the kids all right?

It may seem strange for a book like this to engage with this question as it nears its conclusion. Yet the question speaks to the crux of why it is necessary to argue for a liberal public health in the first place. Shaping a healthier world is fundamentally about the next generation. It is work we do on behalf of those who will inherit the world, and it is work we do in partnership *with* those heirs, as the rising generation increasingly takes its place within the field of public health. The values we embrace are the values that will shape its experience in the years to come. If we do not advance a liberal vision of public health, we do a disservice to the next generation, increasing the likelihood that the kids will not, in fact, be all right. It is up to all of us to ensure that the next generation is supported as it works at shaping a better future.

The young have already done much to support a vision of a healthier world. They have marched, voted, and taken part in the public conversation toward the goal of radically reshaping our society. This engagement has grown considerably. Taking just the example of electoral politics, there was a significant uptick in youth engagement in the 2020 election compared with the 2018 election. After the 2018 election, 33 percent of youth reported attempting to get their peers to vote, and 11 percent reported registering new voters. Months before the 2020 election, 50 percent of youth reported attempting to persuade peers to vote, and 25 percent reported helping to register voters.

This increased engagement appears to be in part a response to the perceived shortcomings of previous generations in creating a better society. This is particularly true in the case of climate change, where the actions—or more accurately inaction—of earlier generations have contributed to a crisis that threatens the health of the entire planet. There is a sense among younger activists that much of their task is to clean up the mess left by those who came before, and this sense underlies the dialogue between the more political members of the younger generation and their elders.

Given these dynamics, and their relevance to the way we address issues of core importance to health, it seems well within the purview of this book to tackle the question of whether the kids are indeed all right, and how the extent to which they may not be all right reflects a broken status quo around issues that matter for a liberal vision of health.

All of us—younger and older—live in a world that is evolving, complex. This reflects a range of fast-moving changes, from the emergence of new technologies, to the advance of social movements, to sudden shocks like political disruptions and the pandemic. Those of us who are old enough to remember what the world was like before this moment are perhaps more apt to fear what all these changes might mean for the future. This fear can cause us to miss the opportunities of the present, the chances urging us to envision a world that is not only better, but radically so. We may also turn to illiberalism out of fear. Those who are younger lack this experience of prior context—this moment of change is their primary reference point in life. They are native to the transitions we see. This status can give them the capacity to notice opportunities older generations miss, and to boldly seize the chance to shape a better world.

This boldness can, of course, have drawbacks. The zeal to shape a better world can at times lead to devaluing what is good about the world we already have. An evolving moral consciousness can prompt a willingness to cast aside much that is useful and necessary from the past. And impatience to get to a better world can cause us to neglect core liberal principles in our rush to end injustice. We are all susceptible to these mistakes, but the young may be at greater risk. They have had, on balance, less exposure to the consequences of pursuing, with maximum certainty, ideas that may be partially formed or wrong. The corrective to this is, of course, experience, as well as the presence of mentors to help the young channel their conviction into an engagement with the world that is fundamentally constructive. Far from being pedantic, this engagement is good for all participants. It gives the young access to valuable advice, and it keeps their elders in dialogue with the future, through those who will one day shape it.

Such a dialogue strikes me as the most effective way of ensuring that the kids—and older generations—remain all right, and invested in a liberal framework. Fundamentally, we are best served by a balance of generational perspectives. By striking this balance, the generations can maximize their strengths and minimize their exposure to pitfalls. Those who are younger can help those who are older better see how the world might be changed at the structural level, by creating a new status quo that is more supportive of health. And older adults can help the young recognize that, in our pursuit of positive change, we need not reinvent everything that has come before—we can draw on the best of past traditions to support an ever-better future.

This balance intersects with the broader project of pursuing a healthier world within a liberal context. The excesses of the younger and of the older, if unchecked, can both lead to forms of illiberal thinking. Those who are younger can be captured by a zeal to rearrange systems, throwing some rather necessary babies out with the bathwater. These include core liberal norms that can look to the young like reactionary roadblocks. Older populations, for their part, in their fear of change, may risk embracing some genuinely reactionary, illiberal notions. These populations can align with political movements that seek to make the future merely an image of the past. Within the field, it is our responsibility to ensure that the rising generation of public health professionals does not fall into the traps we have encountered—from the politicizing of science and public health institutions, to forgetting our roots, to becoming poor at weighing tradeoffs, to losing ourselves in media feedback loops, to cultivating influence rather than pursuing truth. Conversation between the generations, unfolding in a liberal context of respect and civility, can help us avoid these excesses and perhaps even open the door to greater wisdom for everybody. Such conversations also allow older generations to welcome the young to engage with the issues and responsibilities that constitute the pursuit of a better world.

Before concluding, a note by way of full disclosure: in addition to being dean of a school of public health, a position that gives me a daily perspective on the rising generation, I am also the father of two Gen Zers. This has admittedly instilled in me a bias in favor of the younger generation, well positioned as I am to see their commitment to a better world and to recognize how their criticism of past generations is in many ways correct. At the same time, being a parent underscores that those who are younger, however engaged they may be, are still, well, young. There is much they have yet to experience, and this lack of experience can equate to a lack of the hard-won wisdom that comes only through years of living. So it is not responsible to say we should be led by the young in all cases, only that we should listen, always, to the perspective of those who are younger as well as of those who are older, and not patronize or condescend to either group as they contribute to our shared pursuit of a better world, guided by liberal means.

SOURCES

Galea, S. "Public Health and Tradition." *Healthiest Goldfish* (blog), November 19, 2021. https://sandrogalea.substack.com/p/public-health-and-tradition. Accessed April 29, 2022.

Gillard, J. "The 2,500-Year-Old History of Adults Blaming the Younger Generation." History Hustle. https://historyhustle.com/2500-years-of-people-complaining-about-the-younger -generation/. Published April 17, 2018. Accessed April 29, 2022.

McAndrew, J. "New Poll: Young People Energized for Unprecedented 2020 Election." *Tufts Now*, June 30, 2020. https://now.tufts.edu/2020/06/30/new-poll-young-people-energized -unprecedented-2020-election. Accessed April 29, 2022.

Misra, S. "Gen Z Is Calling Millennials Uncool in a New War. Boomers Can Relax Now." *Print*, February 21, 2021. https://theprint.in/opinion/pov/gen-z-is-calling-millennials -uncool-in-a-new-war-boomers-can-relax-now/609001/. Accessed April 29, 2022.

Respectfully Quoted: A Dictionary of Quotations, 1989. Bartleby. https://www.bartleby.com /73/195.html. Accessed April 29, 2022.

In Conclusion

Final thoughts on the road ahead.

TOWARD A LIBERAL
PUBLIC HEALTH

I don't make any of the arguments in these chapters lightly. In the past I have written books and articles making the case for approaches that public health might adopt to shape a healthier world. They were offered as suggestions that public health could take or leave but that I hoped would be adopted, building on past progress to achieve a better future. These writings, then, reflected stakes that were high but not necessarily existential for our field. This book is not like that. I am writing now because I believe that public health is at an inflection point and that to continue down our current path risks seriously compromising our effectiveness. The five problems this book has engaged with—the politicizing of science and public health institutions, forgetting our roots, becoming poor at weighing trade-offs, getting caught in media feedback loops, and cultivating influence rather than pursuing truth—reflect the challenge of this moment. Deciding whether to address these issues is a choice that will shape the future of public health. If we turn a blind eye to the illiberalism in our field, if we do not address the ways we have strayed from our core values, not only will we be unable to support health, we risk actively harming it.

The consequences of an illiberal public health are, to my thinking, threefold. First is the continued marginalizing of our field. I do not mean among policymakers, nor do I mean among those who inhabit the elite institutional spaces where we remain influential. I mean among the general public—our core constituency—who have already lost much trust in us. In our efforts to maintain power and influence, we risk alienating the populations we serve. If this happens it will greatly curtail our capacity to support the health of these populations, undercutting the central function of our field.

Second, illiberalism in public health threatens the future of health science. As I have discussed, science rests on a foundation of reasoned inquiry, a tradition supported by small-*l* liberalism. When science is no longer practiced in a liberal context, it becomes vulnerable to the corrupting influence of politics, ideology, and financial interest. This risks undermining our capacity to generate the knowledge and data that are crucial to the health of populations.

Third, an illiberal public health takes actions that may be morally suspect. I have always believed that public health is a noble profession, but it has had its darker moments when it has perpetrated abuses, often in the name of "the greater good." We now see such moments as aberrations, times when we strayed from our core values. But if these values change, if they are no longer informed by the concerns of small-*l* liberalism, there is little to check what we might do when we decide the moment calls for it, even when the actions being considered are morally questionable. This is a disturbing possibility, one that may be hard for us to consider. But it is also, in many ways, the logical end point of a public health that compromises on its values and turns toward illiberalism.

Suppose we do, in fact, give up on a liberal public health and become fully authoritarian in our methods. What might this look like? We need not search far for the answer. During the pandemic, China took just such an approach to COVID-19. It used the full force of state coercion and mass surveillance to enforce draconian lockdowns that dramatically slowed the spread of the disease, in pursuit of a "zero COVID" strategy. China showed that we can indeed achieve much in the way of stopping disease if we are willing to give up any pretense of protecting civil liberties or valuing liberalism in the pursuit of health. But we can do so only as long as completely eliminating the disease in question seems feasible. The moment it does not—an unavoidable moment, given the nature of infectious disease and the imperfection of human endeavor—crisis can strike. This has happened in China. As I write, COVID is once again surging there, in the country's worst outbreak since the early days of the pandemic. China has responded yet again with strict lockdowns, but its zero-COVID goals are proving elusive, and the government is failing to fully support the populations under lockdown. In Shanghai, for example, emotions boiled over as citizens were heard screaming from their windows in an unsettling display of anger and frustration in the face of food shortages and restrictions on movement.

At the heart of these measures is the implicit belief that the end justifies the means. It is this belief that creates space for ethically dubious measures we would not otherwise consider. China's draconian approach to COVID fits well within an "ends justify the means" rubric, in which the desirable goal of eliminating a disease is used to justify extraordinary, illiberal measures. In the United States public health has done nothing nearly so drastic, but we have sown the seeds of such measures. When we do not have honest, data-informed conversations about the pros and cons of giving a new vaccine to young children, when we shut down good faith debates about lockdown policy, when we ignore the harms such policies can do to vulnerable populations, what are we doing if not starting down a road that can lead to some truly illiberal places?

In writing this book, I hope to reach those in public health who might not have noticed the illiberalism of recent years, to help them see where our field seems to be going and why our course might need correction. But I recognize there are some who may indeed have noticed, and who to some degree approve of, the presence of illiberalism in public health. It is possible to be uncomfortable with illiberalism yet to accept it within public health out of a belief that illiberal means can still deliver healthy populations. Perhaps such means can indeed deliver these results—at least in the short term. But in any embrace of illiberalism there comes a point when the illiberalism becomes not the means but the end, something pursued for its own sake, and the means become our continued self-justification, our defense of the indefensible. We see this in much of China's response to COVID, which has come to seem increasingly irrational, becoming ever more draconian as the goal of zero COVID slips further out of reach.

One of the most troubling aspects of China's approach to the pandemic is that it was endorsed by so many in public health, for whom zero COVID long remained the only acceptable approach to the pandemic. This reflects one of two misunderstandings—or willful oversights. The first concerns the fact that such a goal is in practice impossible. That China, with the country's draconian lockdowns, failed to achieve it should be a lesson to us all. Second, the pursuit of zero COVID requires an authoritarian overreach that we in public health should not allow ourselves to become comfortable with. That so many in our field did not see these points is cause for concern. That so many *did* see them and simply did not care is potentially catastrophic if we do not recognize the strain of illiberalism this reflects and work to mitigate it. When we stop trying to strike a balance between civil liberties and disease prevention, we not only alienate the public, we forget a core fact of health—that it exists to enable a rich, full life. A policy aimed at eliminating all risk at the price of everything that makes life worth living is not a hill we should be willing to die on. And just as we should not embrace such a crackdown, we should not embrace the illiberalism that underlies it.

I wrote this book not from a place of condemnation, but from a place of understanding. The problems public health seeks to solve are significant and structural. In the best of times, working to address them can be a slow, frustrating grind. In moments of crisis such as COVID, endorsing some measure of illiberalism can be tempting as a way of evening the odds. It is not surprising that we chose this path. Fortunately, it isn't too late for us to change course.

The COVID moment was in many ways public health's finest hour. Yet it also created within our field the imaginative space for some truly illiberal approaches. It brought to the surface much that was perhaps always there but was naively overlooked by those who, like me, thought public health was more committed to a liberal framework than it really was. Having glimpsed our darker side, it is now time for us to recommit to a liberal vision for a healthier world. This means recommitting to open inquiry and debate, rejecting undue partisanship, and refusing to adopt policies that require draconian enforcement. Instead, we should accept a realistic engagement with the trade-offs involved in balancing health with the basic liberties of the populations we serve. A liberal public health favors humility instead of certainty, truth instead of power, compassion instead of condemnation. These are the values that have long animated our field, and they have brought us far, allowing us to make tremendous gains in improving the health of populations. As we approach a post-COVID era, these values can again help us advance a vision of a healthier world, win back the trust we have lost, and meet the demands of a moment when the work of public health is more important than ever.

SOURCES

Ferguson, N. "China's 'Zero Covid' Has Become Xi's Nemesis." *Bloomberg*, April 17, 2022. https://www.bloomberg.com/opinion/articles/2022-04-17/china-coronavirus-outbreak -xi-jinping-s-covid-zero-is-failing. Accessed April 29, 2022.

Yuan, L. "China's 'Zero Covid' Mess Proves Autocracy Hurts Everyone." *New York Times*, April 13, 2022. https://www.nytimes.com/2022/04/13/business/china-covid-zero -shanghai.html. Accessed April 29, 2022.

ACKNOWLEDGMENTS

Over the past several years I have had the enormous privilege of working with a team of close colleagues and friends whose passion for the ideas discussed here matches my own. Much of what is in this book emerged from conversations with Eric DelGizzo, Catherine Ettman, and Meredith Brown. Eric brings to this work commitment to the principles that animate what we do, a "sleeves rolled up" engagement with the text, and an attention to detail that makes sure we get it right. This work would be infinitely poorer without his work. Thank you. Catherine has long believed in these ideas and encouraged me to push them forward even—and particularly—during challenging times. She brought indispensable discipline to our team, ensuring that the ideas actually became a book, on schedule. Meredith has always made sure we are delivering on what we promise, even while balancing our full set of responsibilities in the day-to-day realm outside the world of ideas. To all of them, thank you.

Many of the ideas in this book initially appeared in a blog called *The Healthiest Goldfish*. Readers often commented, sharpening the thoughts I first ventured there. I am grateful to all who have engaged with these ideas as they were taking shape. A note of gratitude to Chad Zimmerman, who has long supported my evolution in writing, helping me bridge the gap between ideas and books and making that work enjoyable.

Finally, I have been fortunate to continue my day job while also writing books and papers—I am grateful to all my colleagues at Boston University who make that possible.

INDEX